NO LYE!

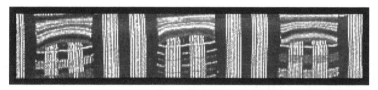

TULANI KINARD

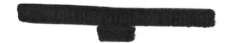

St. Martin's Griffin

New York

Design by Judith Stagnitto Abbate

Illustrations by Mary Greer Mudiku
Photos by Preston Phillips

ISBN 0-312-15180-2

First St. Martin's Griffin Edition: September 1997
10   9   8   7   6   5   4   3   2   1

I DEDICATE THIS BOOK to all of my sisters and brothers who:

- Dare to declare their heads to be a sacred place
- Honor and celebrate their natural beauty
- Walk with regal movement
- See reflections of their light in their children's eyes

May the ase of my mother Osun flow like a warm waterfall sweetened with honey, bathing your ori/consciousness in wisdom, health, beauty, love, truth, prosperity, and sensuality.

ACKNOWLEDGMENTS

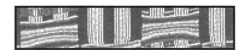

I HAVE SO MUCH to be grateful for. I thank God for answering my requests at every step of my creative process. My family and friends have been wonderful in giving total, unswerving support and unconditional love. I am so grateful for the support and ancestral apprenticeship with Nawili Ayo; her brilliance set the standard. To Iyanla Vanzant, thank you for your love, ase, open arms, and having always said yes from the beginning.

To my husband, Stanley Kinard, beloved, you are the wind beneath my wings. To my children Sakeenah and Alade Kinard, you are the reasons why I fly. Thank you for letting me go whenever I need to. To my mother, Rosalind Jordan, and grandmother Catherine Bramble, thank you for your love and for constantly raising my potential. To my father, Alfred Jordan, thank you for your love and support.

To Bernice Johnson Reagon, thank you for your love, ase, and support.

To Gemmia Vanzant, thank you for covering my back, all the time!

To Alex Morgan, thank you for stepping to my need just in time.

To Mary Greer Mudiku, thank you for your love and ancestral memory.

To my sisters, Valerie Jordan, Jaqueline Kinard, Joy Thompson, Veronica Sealey, Kristen Jordan. To my brother Stephen Jordan, your love and support continues to lift me!

To Avion Julien and Nicole James, of Tulani's Regal Movement, your love and support continue to affirm the fact that "I'm livin' right!" May God give you all you need and desire! You have been, and continue to be, blessings in my life.

To Esmerelda Simmonds, thank you for your love, clarity, and support.

To Maggie Ince, thank you for your love, your home, and the river.

To Suzanne Douglas, thank you for the love and commitment.

Debra Hare-Bey, Cecelia Hinds, Ademola Mandela, Dr. JoAnne Cornwell, Katherine Jones, Leasa Farrar-Fortune, Jeannette Gadson, Gail Baptiste, Halima Taha, Roberta Uno, Shaquisha Coleman, Iyanla Barbara Kenyatta and Chief Bey, and Ile Omo Olofi: thank you for your love and ase.

To Iyalorisa Sabrina and Baba Stephen Parham, thank you for your ase, love, and support.

Iya Joanna Hunter-Mann, thank you for your ase, love, and support.

Awo Adeleri Olayinka, Iya Daria Graham, Baba Craig Brown, thank you for your love and ase.

To my agent, Denise Stinson, thank you for your support and a new beginning.

To my editor, Heather Jackson, thank you for your support and vision. You're one of the chosen few.

Keeley Robinson, thank you for your love and support.

And to Dr. Fred Robinson and Joseph Larayae, thank you for waiting and believing.

Also, thanks go to these people for their contributions:

To Teg Edwards, Master barber . . . in the family, thank you for your support and artistry!!

To Imani Jewelers of New York City, thank you for your elegant creations on the ears of our models.

To Anthony Jones, Brooklyn, and Clavdia, Queens, thank you for your creative excellence in providing the makeup artistry for our models.

To Nilajah Yarborough, your artistry as a natural hair cutter, committed to excellence and style, continues to provide alternatives and nurturing to those who sit in your chair. . . . Peace and Love!

To Debra Hare-Bey, Red Salon, Brooklyn, your commitment to excellence and promotion of the beauty of natural hair care has enriched thousands of lives. As a colleague, and friend your support and love has stood the test of time. Thank you, Genique!

To Ademola Mandela, Locs and Chops Salon, New York. As an elder in this industry, you have inspired the masses with an African-centered style, regal elegance, and funk that has crossed the barriers of gender and age. As a colleague and friend your support and love throughout the years continues to validate the reasons why we do what we do!

To Preston Phillips. Truth be told . . . your lens has documented most of the master natural hair care artists of the past decade in New York, and you continue to do so. . . . Your support and love of our ancestrally inspired hair sculptures will serve to reveal to our children and for generations to come, the revolutionary process of the healing and transformation of Kings and Queens! Modupe (thank you).

My deepest appreciation goes to the women, men, children, and their parents who gave of their time, wonderful energy, and love to ensure the success of this book: Suzzanne Douglas, Iyanla Vanzant, Lailah Callaway, Muntu Doggett-Law, Luther Williams, Chandra Dunmars, Amma McKen, Esmerelda Simmons, Stanley Kinard, Amma Fruster, Caren Calder, Debra Green, Sabrina Parham, Wendy Mahdi, Monette Russell-Ward, Shakesha Coleman, Tracy

Titus, Imani Cummings, Talida Edwards, Sakeenah Kinard, Arlene Joseph, Ola Ellis, Gabrielle Hawkins, Alade Kinard, Osaremi Parham, Olatunde Spellman, Alexandra McCain, and Sinead Stewart.

To the designers and boutiques that make life on the road a beautiful thing. . . . Modupe: Rosalind Jordan, Boston; and in New York City—Brenda Brunson-Bey and Zawadi of 4W Circle, Jamila's, Nyota Muhammad of Tents of Kedar, Phati of Sankofa Creations, Yvonne James, Ademola, Owa African Market, Marva Lane, Malik Tall, Moshood, and Status.

CONTENTS

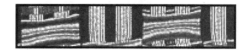

INTRODUCTION

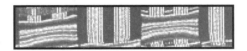

I T WAS IN THE FALL OF 1978 in Washington, D.C., and I just had my hair braided for the first time by a sister named Sherifu. Shea, as she was affectionately called by those in D.C.'s cultural community, was from Los Angeles. Her work reflected what was known as an "L.A. vibe," in that it was totally artistic, full of precision, and loaded with elegance. When I looked in the mirror, I saw that a total transformation had taken place. I started crying and laughing at the same time. I was elated. A mixture of joy, familiarity, beauty, and a sense of peace came over me all at once. My soul was rejoicing.

I left her house and chose to walk home instead of taking the bus, because I was so excited. As I walked down Rhode Island Avenue, old and young men, children, and women of all ages complimented me. Their accolades about my hair ranged from approving grunts and moans to actually stopping to inspect, question, and give praise to Shea's hair sculpture on my head.

Even though I had worn my hair in an Afro for most of my life, every now and then the urge to have "bouncin' and behavin'" hair would creep up on me. You would think that nearly going bald within a month of having my hair permed at a reputable salon would truly have been enough to convince me never to embrace a Eurocentric style of hair design again in my life, but it wasn't. My experience on Rhode Island Avenue definitely did the trick.

Soon thereafter, another L.A.-based braider come to town and took me to another realm. Nawili Ayo, who carried the title of Queen of the Itty Bitty Braids, braided my hair in microbraids and adorned them with jewels of semiprecious stones and crystals. Whenever I went out, the compliments and approval for my hairstyle never stopped. It became a truly humbling experience for me.

At the same time, I felt charged with another level of energy, only adding to the regalness and confidence I acquired when I first had my hair braided.

In moments of quiet self-reflection, I realized I had never before received such a sincere outpouring of appreciation for my beauty. I felt love and support from strangers of different races, genders, and age groups. It was a very powerful experience. It made me feel beautiful, self-confident, and totally aware of the power of an African aesthetic. These African-American women who had braided my hair had not traveled to Africa, yet they were inspired to create these ancestrally charged hair sculptures.

Since then I have worn many different natural hair sculptures. I believe the transmission of all of that creative energy to my head served to make me aware of my calling. So under the tutelage of Nawili Ayo, I learned the art of braiding.

At that time in my life I was a full-time member of the a cappella singing group Sweet Honey in the Rock. One evening while performing, I literally lost my voice. After seeking medical advice about my vocal condition, I was given the choice of either having surgery performed on my vocal chords or going for an extended period of time in total vocal silence. So I chose silence as my path to recovery.

The silence of my voice made room for the hand-sung expressions of beauty, whose origins connected me to ancestral realms and awakened my consciousness.

As my fingers caressed each person's head, I felt good about creating a beautiful hairstyle without altering the natural texture of the hair. I realized that caring for our hair without harsh chemicals—natural hair care—is the only way for it to be truly healthy. Through applying what I've learned about natural hair care, I've witnessed a total rejuvenation of damaged hair that would otherwise have been doomed.

We shun natural hair care because we have been told for generations that "nappy" hair is bad and made to feel that the only way to attain "good" hair is to straighten it "by any means necessary." As we approach the next millennium, many things are being revealed about the products we use, the foods we eat, and the overall conditions that leave many of us in a diseased state. As a healer and teacher I cannot sit back, say nothing, and accept what I know to be destructive to our hair—and to our self-esteem I am blessed with the opportunity to share my experiences with you as well as guide you along the path to natural hair care.

Over the past fifteen years, I have seen a large number of people with chemically damaged heads of hair. What I've seen is only a small percentage of a much greater number of people who've nearly destroyed their hair's natural beauty through these harsh processes. While a student in cosmetology school, I witnessed many men and women requesting that chemical straighteners be applied to their already severely damaged heads. Upon being informed of the danger of inflicting further damage to their hair, often the response was, "Well, what am I supposed to do?" or "It'll grow back." The desire for "bone straight" hair ("good hair") is embedded so deeply in the psyches of so many people that it has become part of African-American cultural experience. By the time a child reaches her teens, more than likely she's already had her hair chemically straightened at least once, if not repeatedly.

It has taken this society twenty-five years to accept African-inspired natural hair sculpting. I would be totally remiss if I did not state that, although the natural-hair-care movement is in good stride, there are many who still feel the effects of racism at the workplace because of the way they wear their hair. (Recently, an article appeared in the *New York Post* that quoted black professionals as saying that they did not feel braids were appropriate for the workplace.) Why are braids so threatening? What inspires this fear? The answer lies in the perception of what is "good" hair—an ingrained misconception that is being turned on its head.

The number of people wearing their hair naturally has increased dramatically. What was once considered a fad is quickly becoming the norm. This is best illustrated by the fact that the media is now portraying these styles—in advertising, on soap operas, in magazines, etc. This movement has created a demand for the services of natural-hair-care specialists, which in turn has created a need for professional accreditation.

In 1989, I wrote the language that defined natural hair care and all its tenets (which included a "grandfather clause for practitioners") in New York. It was this state's first legislative bill for natural hair care. In 1992, with the expertise of civil rights attorney Esmerelda Simmons and the support of state Senator Velmonette Montgomery, New York became the first state in the country to offer and require a natural-hair-care license. It took more than ten years for the Washington, D.C., city council and cosmetology board to accept having a braiding license—in a city whose population is more than 70 percent African American! But, due to the unrelenting struggles of a dedicated few, led by local natural-hair-care specialist Pamela Ferrell and her husband, Talib Din-Uqdah, Washington, D.C., finally adopted a braiding license in 1996. Currently, Washington, D.C. and New York state are the only two places that require natural hair care practitioners to have licenses. Although we have claimed a victory for professional recognition for the art form/industry, there is still an ongoing struggle to amend language and techniques within the legislation that have nothing to do with natural hair care, and everything to do with time and money for those who do not have this industry's best interest at heart. There is intense legislative activity going on in Illinois, California, and Michigan, however. Let this book serve as your hair "bible," your protection until licensing becomes required nationwide.

NO LYE! AT-A-GLANCE

Throughout the book we will:

• Explore the biological composition of black hair, in its variety of textures.
• Give tips to recognizing the essential ingredients that make up a good shampoo and conditioner for whatever hair type you have or state your hair may currently be in. Every woman should know how to purchase products that are nourishing to her hair. The ability to make choices from a place of knowledge will save you time, money, and stress.
• Give a brief historical insight into traditional African influences on the expression of natural hair sculptures.
• In wanting always to provide the best for our children, the book offers an in-depth step-by-step guide to grooming their hair from the cradle to adolescence.
• Locs are hot . . . and you'll learn the ins and outs of one of the most innovative and healthy ways to style and groom your hair.
• The pros and cons of wearing extensions are explored and explained thoroughly. Along with photos of popular braiding styles, we identify the different fibers that are used to create these styles and give step-by-step instruction on correct braiding techniques.
• Go beyond braids, and show you ways you can enhance the beauty of your natural hairstyle.

Eventually your status as an "educated consumer" will have an impact upon the product manufacturer's research-and-development process. You will move away from products that are popular or familiar, toward products that you know will satisfy your hair's biochemical needs. Manufacturers will then be forced to create products based upon your demand for those that are "biochemically correct."

If your hair has been overprocessed and damaged, after reading this book you will have an understanding as to how it happened, what you can do to prevent it from happening in the future, and what you can do to aid in the rejuvenation of your hair.

If you are in the care of a professional stylist (natural-hair-care specialist, cosmetologist, or barber), and up to this point haven't had a clue as to what is going on with your hair, you will now be able to have an intelligent conversation about your hair-care regime.

A word of caution, though: Somebody said that a little knowledge can be a dangerous thing. This is not a doctoral degree program, or an apprenticeship course; however, the simple "how-to" sections are designed to help you become comfortable with the natural texture of your hair. This is a guide to help you, wherever you may be on the path of natural hair care. It helps you not only with aesthetics, but also with scientific information that will allow you to make better choices. For many of you, this will actually be the first time you will receive support for exploring, embracing, and celebrating your natural hair. So take your time. Enjoy the process, and allow yourself to fully experience your natural beauty.

"I live to serve, because I have a charge to keep."

—TULANI KINARD
December 6, 1996

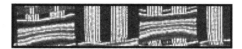

THE ROOT OF IT ALL

THE HAIR THAT COVERS OUR BODIES is separated into three categories: short hairs, lanugo hairs, and long hairs. The body will generate the appropriate thickness and length of hair for whatever area needs its particular protection. The **short hairs** are those on our eyebrows and eyelashes, on our armpits, in our nostrils, and in numerous other places on our bodies. These hairs serve to protect sensitive areas of our skin. **Lanugo hair** is very soft, downy "baby" hair. Infants are born with this type of hair covering their bodies in various places, such as their ears, arms, and legs. As they grow older the body naturally sheds this hair. **Long hair** grows from the scalp. It serves to protect the head from injury, and from the elements—the sun, cold weather, etc. The length to which this hair will grow is already predetermined by the DNA in the body.

We are constantly exposed to an onslaught of commercials and other advertisements claiming to be "just the product your hair needs to be healthy, long, and luxurious." For clarity's sake, there is no product that is going to make your hair grow long. The length of your hair is determined by your genes. There are products, however, that can aid the sheen, strength, and overall well-being of your hair—once you understand its biochemical makeup. Get ready to enjoy the freedom of knowing what products best serve you and your hair type.

DON'T GET STRANDED: UNDERSTAND YOUR HAIR'S COMPOSITION

The name for the strand of hair *after* it emerges from the scalp is **keratin.** The biochemical name for hair *before* it emerges from the skin is **follicle.** (We'll refer to it as hair follicle just to keep the relation clear.) **Hair follicles** are composed of hydrogen, oxygen, carbon, sulfur, and phosphorus.

The skin plays a very important role in the growth and development of the hair follicle, so an understanding of skin's "makeup" is important. The top layer of skin that we see, touch, and feel is called the **dermis;** it has seven layers. At the bottom of these layers is the **epidermis.** This is where all of the nerves, blood vessels, smooth muscles, sweat glands, and **sebaceous glands** (oil glands) develop and grow.

Deep within the epidermis, nerves, blood vessels, and a great supply of blood form into a thick, bulb shape called the **papilla.** The papilla is covered with cells that are 90 percent water, which is why moisture is so very important for our hair. The follicle, a narrow, tubular-shaped cell, takes root in the papilla and grows upward through the layers of skin, while attached to the sebaceous gland. Any disease or injury that destroys the papilla or follicle will stop the hair from growing in that area. Inside each follicle are three layers of cells. The inner core of these layers is the **medulla,** the middle layer is the **cortex,** and the outer layer is the **cuticle.** Not much is known about the function of the medulla. However, it is known that the medulla is not present in the lanugo hairs.

Certain laboratory tests can be performed on the medulla to as-

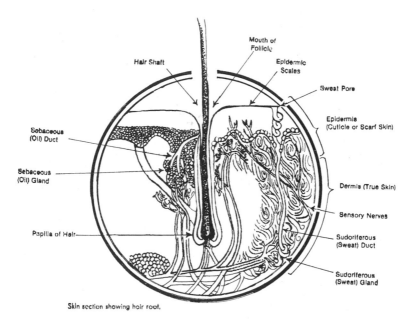

Skin section showing hair root.

The inner structure of skin and hair (curly hair strand). *(Illustration by Mary E. Mudiku)*

sess your diet and drug-use history; this information is stored within the core of the hair follicle. The second layer is the cortex. Its fibers determine the strength and elasticity of the hair follicle. The cortex contains melanin. Melanin is the substance that causes pigmentation, and determines the color of our hair and skin. The more melanin present in the cortex, the darker your hair and skin will be.

The fibers in the cortex are very sensitive to chemicals and can be easily damaged by the chemicals used in hair straighteners, hair dyes, and some shampoos.

The outer layer of the follicle, the cuticle, is composed of microscopic thin layers of scales that lie on top of one another. Cuticles determine the porosity of the hair, or your hair's absorption ability. They open and close like window shutters or blinds. Extremely tight, curly African, Asian, and Hispanic hair have many

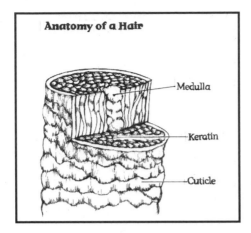

Anatomy of a Hair

Medulla

Keratin

Cuticle

The structure of the hair follicle. *(Illustration by Mary E. Mudiku)*

more layers of cuticles than straight European hair. The cuticles' microscopic scales serve as protection to the cortex and the medulla. Cuticles can be opened with a key that fits, like a shampoo with the chemical balance (pH factor) that your hair needs, or they can be opened like a SWAT-team attack, as with a chemical relaxer.

Now that we have described the hair follicle, there is one more important factor in the growth and development of a healthy head of hair: the sebaceous gland. It is attached to the follicle, and does not become exposed to the surface of the skin, staying imbedded in the epidermis. This gland is responsible for producing the oil that lubricates the scalp and the hair follicle as it emerges through the dermis. The sebaceous gland is directly affected by any change in your diet, by poor blood circulation, emotional disturbances, and any type of drug use.

As the hair follicle grows up and penetrates the dermis, it takes on a new shape, and two new names. The air causes it to oxidize (it becomes hard) and turns it into a protein substance called keratin. The physical structure of this follicle is the **hair shaft** or **hair strand** (they mean the same thing).

The size of an average head is about 120 square inches, and there are about 1,000 strands of hair per square inch, giving the average head about 120,000 strands of hair. The average rate of growth of a strand of hair is ½ inch per month, and up to 7 or 8 inches per year. Now, one would think that if your head were a few inches smaller in diameter you would have less hair. Or that if it were a few inches larger you would have more hair. In fact, the amount of hair a person has is actually determined by the texture and color of the hair. The naturally blond-haired person has an average of 140,000 hairs, the natural brunette about 110,000 strands, and natural redheads average 90,000 strands.

SHAPE UP: DETERMINING YOUR HAIR'S SHAPE

There are basically three shapes the follicle can take when it is forming in the papilla: curly, wavy, or straight. When the curly follicle emerges from the dermis, the shape of the hair shaft is flat. The wavy follicle is oval in shape, and the straight follicle is round (these shapes are not visible to the naked eye; they can only be seen under a microscope).

The textures of these shapes are fine, medium, and coarse. Texture is determined by the overall diameter of the hair strand. The coarser the hair texture, the more voluminous the hair will be. The hair strand's diameter is determined by whether or not the medulla is present (remember, earlier we said that it's not present in fine "lanugo" hair), how large the cortex is, and/or how many layers of the cuticle are packed on top of one another. Coarse hair has the largest diameter and fine hair has the smallest, with medium texture right in the middle of the two. Within our race, due to interracial ancestry, these aforementioned natural shapes and textures take on many different genetic combinations. To keep it simple, we will stick to three general shapes—curly, wavy, and straight—and three textural types: fine, medium, and coarse.

THE LOOK AND FEEL OF IT: DETERMINING YOUR HAIR'S TEXTURE

Examine your hair. How does it feel? What does it look like? Is it short, medium, or long in length? What happens when you pull it away from your scalp and let it drop? Does it fall straight down, recoil or spring back to the scalp, or do something in between?

Would you describe the shape of your hair strand as curly, straight, or wavy? Would you describe its texture as coarse, medium, or fine? The shape of your hair strand could be curly, and your hair texture fine; or you could determine that your hair is wavy and medium-textured.

Fine hair has the smallest diameter of the three texture types when measured, because it does not have a medulla. Because the medulla is not present, the hair strand is lighter and has that "fly-away" feeling. Fine hair can be any length; it is soft to the touch.

Medium hair has a diameter that falls in between coarse and fine-textured hair. It can be any length. The texture would be fairly smooth—not as rough as coarse hair, nor as soft as fine hair.

Coarse hair can be any length. It feels rough to the touch. The coarse hair strand has the largest diameter (width) of all the hair textures, and it has many cuticle layers. Coarse hair can be very curly or wavy. Straight, coarse hair usually has some kind of wave pattern to it, because its many cuticle layers cause the hair strand to bend. (However, it does not bend to the point where you would classify it as wavy hair.) The diameter of the coarse strand will not look much bigger to the naked eye, but under a microscope the cuticle layers will become visible, and its size will become more apparent when compared to medium and fine hair strands.

TEXTURE TEST

To determine your hair texture, take this simple test. If you get a friend to take it at the same time, most of the differences are visible to the naked eye.

Pull out a strand of your hair. Place your index finger and thumb on the strand, then slide them up and down along its length. How does it feel? How does it look? If it feels smooth yet a bit bumpy, and it looks thick, that means it's coarse. Check out your friend's hair, then check out the chart.

We have always thought that because our hair is curly it should be described as coarse or medium, and never fine. I tried the test

TEXTURE CHART

	COARSE	MEDIUM	FINE
STRAIGHT	**Length:** Short, medium, long **Texture:** Rough, wiry★ **Diameter:** Measures the largest due to the layers of cuticles **Weight:** Heavy, dense, thick	**Length:** Short or long **Texture:** Fairly smooth, straight **Diameter:** Average **Weight:** Average	**Length:** Short or long **Texture:** Smooth, soft, straight **Diameter:** Smallest; it has no medulla **Weight:** Lightweight, flyaway, thin
CURLY	**Length:** Short, medium, long **Texture:** Rough, springy★★ **Diameter:** Largest, coiled close to the scalp **Weight:** Heavy, dense, thick	**Length:** Short, medium **Texture:** Soft, springy like cotton **Diameter:** Average, between large and small **Weight:** Average thickness	**Length:** Short, medium, long **Texture:** Smooth **Diameter:** Smallest **Weight:** Light
WAVY	**Length:** Short, medium, long **Texture:** Rough, wiry **Diameter:** Largest, due to layers of cuticles **Weight:** Heavy, dense, thick	**Length:** Short, medium, long **Texture:** Smooth, supple **Diameter:** Average **Weight:** Average	**Length:** Short, medium, and long **Texture:** Very soft **Diameter:** Smallest **Weight:** Light

★ Will not hang straight since heavy layers of cuticle tend to bend, making it wiry
★★ Usually coiled close to the scalp

you just took with a friend of mine. Both our hair is very curly, and it looks the same at first glance. But when we pulled out a strand of our hair, felt them, and laid them side by side, we saw that they were very different.

To our surprise, when we looked at the hair strands, hers was much thicker than mine and could be described as coarse-curly. Mine was fine-curly. Now that you know how to determine the true nature of your hair, you will be better able to take the proper care of it.

CHAPTER
TWO

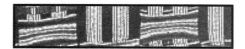

THE BREAKING POINT

SO MANY FOLKS HAVE SUFFERED due to chemical straighteners. When I began my career as a braider, I was very much against women having their hair chemically straightened. I saw so many women suffering from all types of hair loss. Alopecia areata, age, heredity, and stress were some of the most common causes. The cause that seemed at almost epidemic proportions, though, was chemical damage. After a basic introduction to the chemistry of relaxers, I was driven to learn more about how these different products altered the natural texture of our hair. I reviewed the historical development of our history in "beauty culture" and product manufacturing. I was clear about three things:

1. African-American entrepreneurs created a market for products that served the needs of millions of people of color around the world, and were very successful financially.

2. Those entrepreneurs also paved the way for thousands of aspiring "beauticians" to open businesses that created a solid economic base within their communities.

3. Although these businesses were wonderful for economic empowerment and independence, with the exception of barber shops, the *foundation* of beauty salons was the money that flowed from the use of thermal implements and chemicals to alter the natural state of black hair.

The level of damage that occurred to our hair, and the perpetuation of deep psychological denial of our natural beauty, can hardly be ignored. The level of psychological, physical, and even spiritual damage black women have endured to attain an unnatural beauty ideal is incredible. Add to that the physical pain of lye-based products and the embarrassment of losing your hair temporarily or permanently because of the use of chemical straighteners, and the cost is one no woman should have to pay.

The fact of the matter is, the success of these businesses was predicated upon the underlying effects of slavery and racism. The denial of the beauty of our natural hair in order to assimilate into the dominant culture that was responsible for untold atrocities against our people, was more than I could accept. The more I came to understand the strength and toxicity of these products, the more alarmed I became. What's worse, these products were the foundation for most of the popular styles African-American women have been wearing since the 1950s. They not only serve as a reminder of the denial of our natural beauty, but are also a denial of ourselves, our culture, and our history.

WHAT YOUR HAIRDRESSER
MAY NOT TELL YOU

Real work and patience are required in order to bring your hair back to its natural, healthy state. Based upon my research and experience, it is impossible for chemically processed hair to be healthy.

And I'm sorry, but if you have a chemical straightener in your hair, and your stylist is telling you your hair is healthy, know one of two things right away:

1. Your stylist is totally ignorant of the process of maintaining a healthy head or hair and of the biochemical realities of a hair strand; or
2. Your stylist is not being totally honest. (Let me be kind; I have many associates who are cosmetologists. This is not a personal attack.)

They have been perming hair for so long, and doing what they learned in beauty school as the proper way to deal with our hair that this misinformation is now part of their belief systems. These beliefs are slow to change, especially when money and personal livelihood are tied into it.

If you take the time to understand the biochemical makeup of your hair and the damaging properties of these chemical straighteners, I have no doubt that with the use of critical thinking skills, you too will see "the lye."

CHEMICAL STRAIGHTENERS

There are two types of relaxers that serve as the foundation for altering the genetic pattern of a strand of hair. They are **sodium hydroxide** and **ammonium thioglycolate.**

Sodium hydroxide is very high on the pH factor scale, a highly alkaline product. It can cause permanent damage when used incorrectly, and some level of damage even when used correctly. That's just the way it is. This product is lye-based. It is used to straighten the hair. There will be no curl pattern. The effects of this type of chemical straightener cannot be reversed. It is said that this type of relaxer doesn't dry out the hair strand as much as the ammonium thioglycolate product, but I have never seen a naturally moisturized, chemically processed head of hair. When these chemical

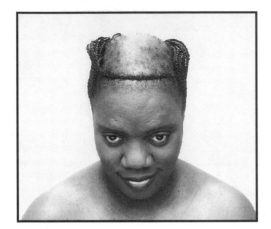

Chandra's hair has suffered from a combination of alopecia and permanent chemical damage. She is blessed in that she still has hair around the sides and back of her head. This small amount of hair has enabled the stylist to create a cornrow sculpture that will cover the damaged area.

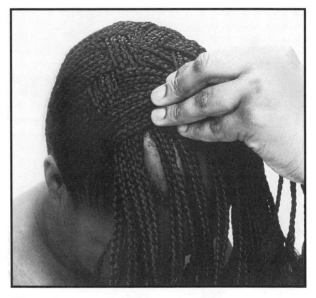

The ends of the cornrow extensions have been braided down to provide a means to create a basket weave effect.

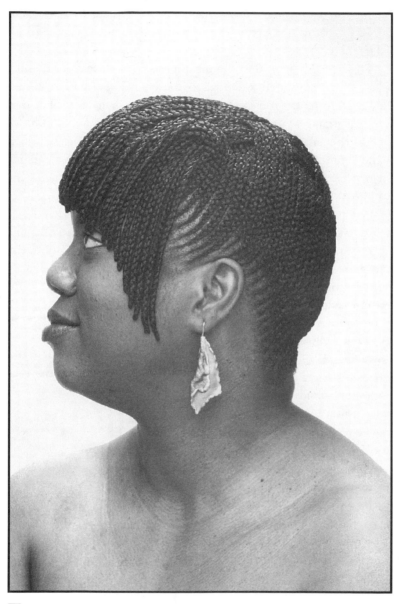

The braids are then sewn together into a secure bang, leaving the alopecia area totally undetectable. We are eternally grateful to Chandra for sharing her condition. We hope it inspires others to seek braided sculptures as a natural alternative to wearing a wig. *(Hair sculpture, Nicole James)*

straighteners are applied to the hair, they immediately work against moisture, because any retention of it would reduce their rate of effectiveness.

This is why after the chemical process, a deep-conditioning treatment is absolutely essential to the hair. These treatments are designed to return moisture back to the hair shaft, as well as coat the hair strand (as in the case of thio perms, which are also known as curly perms; the curl activator and moisturizer try to achieve the same result). Chemical straighteners will guarantee you a lifetime of dry hair and scalp. They walk hand in hand. It's a marriage—and one that's bound to "break" up.

If you want to wear a style that requires a curl, you'll need heat for quick results. Rolling and setting the hair to create curls, and sitting under a hot dryer to set the curl is commonplace. But in this day and age, who has the time to sit under a dryer with a roller set waiting for it to dry? That is what you should do to minimize damage. The dryer at a low temperature is definitely the lesser of a few evils when it comes to styling chemically straightened hair. But alas, the setting lotion also tends to rob your hair of moisture. The maintenance regime you must use to look stylish after a perm—i.e., sitting under a hot dryer; thermal curling of the hair, and blow-drying—are tried-and-true ways on the path to thin hair for some, and a bald head for others.

The prevailing trend of not adding oil to the hair or scalp (because it weighs the hair down) to create a light

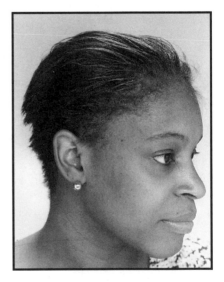

Wendy has suffered from damage due to the over-processing of her hair. Her hairline is just about gone, and what is left of it is very frail.

"bouncin' and behavin'" look is also another way to support dry conditions on the scalp and hair shaft. Why does hair break? No moisture. The natural oils your body produces can't serve your hair's needs, because of your steady regimen of touch-ups (perms, curling irons, etc.) to maintain "the look." So after a period of time—short for some, a little longer for others—the need for a cut to camouflage the damage done to your hair will become your signature style.

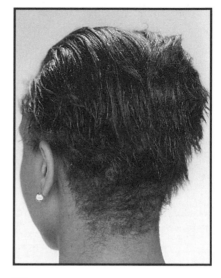

The back has broken off so badly, previously the only solution would be to get a fade cut.

When that "designer cut" (like *the fade*) is suggested, it should be the cue that your hair has truly had enough, and needs TLC: Totally Lye-free Care.

THE TRUTH ABOUT THIO

The ammonium thioglycolate products ("thios") have three claims to fame: (1) they are used for sensitive scalps; (2) they are milder than sodium hydroxide—lye-based products; and (3) "best of all," you can go directly from a thio straightening relaxer into a thio-based curl perm—a double whammy for your already damaged hair.

The results of thio-based relaxers are similar to those of the sodium hydroxide relaxers. The chemical bonding is very different, however. These two products cannot be used together. Let me explain so you have total clarity. You cannot go from having a sodium hydroxide "straight" relaxer to a thioglycolate "curl." Your hair would probably melt right in your hands. You must also be careful of using "no lye" products when changing from one product to the next. Some of these products contain sodium bromide, which is very similar to sodium hydroxide.

Again, you cannot stop using a thio-based product and just change over to a no-lye product. Your hair will experience severe damage. Even though thio-based products are not as harsh as sodium hydroxide products, they also strip your hair of moisture. Clear evidence of this are the thio-based "curl" products. They gave new meaning to "bouncin' and behavin'."

When I attended cosmetology school, women would come to receive hair-care services for a nominal fee from the school's students. At the time, the "curly perm" was in "full effect." People were marveling over the fact that not only was their hair growing, but it was soft and curly, too! You could have this new look with little or no hair, even if your hair was damaged. There were rod sizes for every little piece of hair. I witnessed students not using gloves, because it would slow them down. My hands were everything to me, so I wore at least two pairs of gloves. I wanted to wear the big yellow gloves, but I was discouraged because it would scare the clients. But in reality I wanted to ask them, "Would you put this cream on your face—or better, on your arm, and leave it there for just half of the recommended time?" I don't think so. Then why would anyone put this on their heads? The skin absorbs everything, and as strong as the chemical is—causing sores and abrasions on the scalp—why wouldn't some of it seep through the skull and into the brain? Given the basic facts and logic of how the body works, there is no way anyone could convince me that such a strong chemical product is not leaving some kind of residue in the bloodstream, at the very least.

Everyone believed the "curl" really "grew some hair." In fact, it thinned and dried out the hair shaft. The "growth" experienced was the result of new growth coming in, and the hair not being combed in the usual way which gave the appearance of having more hair. Much like a frayed rope end appears thicker and fuller than the rope itself—when indeed it's frail and damaged.

The "curl" moisturizer was essential to keeping the hair from drying out and breaking off right away. After a while, the "curly perm" began to break off because the hair shaft was too thin. This breakage was not noticed right away because it would occur slowly, and it was hidden by the curls and the new growth. I have observed (as with all forms of chemical straighteners) that the actual width of the hair strand becomes thinner—just as the "rope" becomes weaker as the fraying extends down its length.

Eventually, the "curl" moisturizing juice cannot coat the damaged, thin hair strands. Remember the scene in Eddie Murphy's *Coming to America* where the "curl" family left a stain on the couch from the moisturizer dripping off their hair? Well, shawls for the shoulders started appearing at around the same time as "designer" cuts, because the moisturizing-activator products dripped right off the damaged hair strands. In essence, this means the cuticle was so damaged that it could no longer hold any product on the outer layer of the hair shaft. This type of breakage was not obvious to the wearer, because in most cases the new growth gave the illusion of thick hair; it was not until the damage was pervasive that people realized what was going on.

WHEN YOU'VE "GOTTA HAVE IT"

There are beauticians who follow the rule that very curly hair requires a strong perm, left on for a short period of time. They believe stronger works faster, and puts less chemical stress on the hair shaft. What they fail to take into account is the porosity (the ability to absorb) of an individual's hair. There are over fifty different types of natural hair spanning the human race; people of color can account for more than forty of them. Add that fact to the person's prior hair treatment and health status (any hair reaction to medication, vitamins, or drugs), and the need for a mandatory preliminary patch test is obvious.

Realistically, if you've got to have a perm, your hair must be tested to determine its pH factor, curl pattern, texture, density, natural growth patterns, strength of the strand, as well as its porosity before a chemical straightener or color is applied.

But who has time for that? "The fade" will always be around. It's a classic, timeless look. Now you know why!

Just for the record: *No chemically straightened hair can be reverted back to its natural state.* The only option for returning to a natural state is letting the hair grow out naturally, then cutting off the damaged, "straightened" part. No Lye!

ALOPECIA AREATA—PATTERN BALDNESS

Alopecia areata is a form of hair loss that is not restricted by race or gender. There is some research suggesting that pattern baldness is hereditary, and in that situation, the baldness is reportedly more likely to affect a few people in the family. The women and men in the family may thin in the same place, after a certain age. I tend to think that the word *hereditary* applies not only to a genealogical cell structure, but also to a lifestyle and eating patterns that are inherent within a family.

THE GALEA MEMBRANE

In Dr. Pavlo Airola's book *Stop Hair Loss,* there is an extensive discussion on research conducted on male pattern baldness in the 1950s and '60s by the late Dr. Lars Engstrand of the Karolinska Institute in Stockholm, Sweden. Dr. Engstrand conducted research on and successfully treated over one thousand men in various stages of baldness. His research revealed that baldness is caused by pressure on the capillaries (tiny blood vessels) of the scalp caused by the galea (the membrane underneath the scalp). The galea is located on the crown of the head. It covers an area of approximately forty square inches, starting at the lower forehead, going back and along the sides to the earlobes. This is the approximate line where typical complete baldness stops. It also has a growth cycle.

At the age of fifteen, the membrane is paper thin in both men and women. Between the ages of sixteen and eighteen, a man's galea becomes thicker and loses its elasticity. For women, however, it remains elastic throughout life. So, according to this research, women's pattern baldness would be attributable to something other than a thickened galea.

I would also raise serious questions as to the effect of chemical straighteners on the galea membrane. The scalp is skin. Anything that we put on it gets absorbed. It would seem to me that years of applying chemical straighteners, which are acidic and toxic, to the scalp would allow these chemicals to permeate the intracellular structure of the galea.

They could also have some other effects on the body, especially the liver. The liver is an organ that acts as a filter for organic and inorganic matter in the body. It absorbs chemicals, and because of this chemicals can build up in the liver over a period of time, having a direct effect on the skin.

Whenever the skin is traumatized in any way, it is directly connected to the liver. Any damage to the liver will be reflected by the skin. This trauma would also affect the hormonal balance of the papilla. The slightest imbalance in the body can adversely affect the papilla, and in turn the growth of our hair.

There are many areas to consider when embarking upon an investigation into Alopecia.

Medications that may cause alopecia are:
• penicillin, sleeping pills, birth control pills, blood pressure pills, and excessive use of aspirin.

Exposure to large amounts of radiation from:
• chemotherapy, x-rays, radium, atomic accidents and explosions (although hair loss would be the least of your worries).

Applied stress, pulling the hair in a variety of ways is another cause of baldness:

• Securing rollers too tightly, barrettes, bobby pins, rubber bands for pony tails, and braids, can cause temporary or permanent damage to the hair follicles.

Many infections lay at the root of hair loss, such as fungal bacteria (staphylococcal and streptococcal), viral (herpes), or ringworm. Fortunately, if these infections are diagnosed and treated early in their development they can be arrested with medication, thereby preventing permanent hair loss.

There are also a whole host of systemic diseases that can cause baldness. They include: lupus, leukemia, cancer, pituitary disorders, scarlet fever, syphillis, advanced diabetes, and influenza. Drugs or chemicals with toxic effects when ingested or applied to the skin or hair can also cause hair loss.

The thickening of the galea membrane continues for men until the age of fifty to fifty-five. After that it stabilizes and remains unchanged, then begins to thin out. During this time, many elderly men experience new hair growth in areas that were previously bald.

When the galea becomes thick, it increases the pressure and tension on the scalp. This pressure stops the blood from circulating properly, which in turn prevents the papilla from receiving the proper nutrients necessary for it to produce hair. In advanced cases of baldness, the membrane may increase up to ten times its normal size, and will completely block the distribution of blood to the capillaries.

In addition to age, several other factors may cause the galea membrane to thicken and interfere with hair growth. When thinning occurs before the age of twenty-five, it is thought to be hereditary. Dr. Engstrand believed that men who have thickened galeas have them because of overstimulation of—and therefore depletion of—male sex hormones. (Wild men beware! Too much of a good thing may leave you bald.) Taoism (Chinese philosophy) supports the theory that the loss of male sexual hormones and energy will not only thin your hair, but decrease your life expectancy as well. Dr. Engstrand's treatment for pattern baldness consisted of an operation on the scalp to remove some of the galea.

If you have this problem, remember that before adopting any treatment plan you should check with your physician or dermatologist. A knowledgeable, holistically minded doctor will agree that a change in lifestyle, as well as a whole-body approach to this ailment, is a good place to start. Whether or not you have problems of hair loss or thinning, following the advice laid out below is important to your hair's health.

YOU ARE WHAT YOU EAT—
AND SO IS YOUR HAIR!

Since we know hair growth is determined by internal factors—stress, diet, exercise, genetics—getting started on your path to natural hair care requires that you put good things into your body, so that better hair may come out.

FOODS FOR HEALTHIER HAIR

Here is a list of basic, health-promoting whole foods and supplements:

Kale
Spinach
Okra
Collards
Broccoli
Cabbage★
Beans

★Eat raw or cooked, but don't overcook veggies, as their nutrients get depleted the longer they are cooked.

Nuts
Seeds
Legumes
Seafood
Seaweed
Whole grains
Fruits
Plenty of H_2O

VITAMINS AND SUPPLEMENTS

Most vitamin bottles will state what the recommended dosage is for an adult according to the % U.S. RDA standards. If you are interested in taking vitamins specifically designed to nourish the hair, most manufacturers will give a general recommendation of the dosage you should ingest. Careful observation of your hair will let you know whether you should increase or decrease the dosage. (Again check with your doctor before beginning any new diet or supplementation program.)

B complex
Silica
Vitamin C (Rose hip tea is an abundant natural source)
Multivitamin

THINGS TO AVOID

Fatty foods
High-calorie foods
Fried foods
Smoking*
Sugar and processed foods

*Constricts arteries and capillaries, slows circulation

KEEPING BALDNESS AT BAY

In addition to leading a healthier lifestyle, here are some other natural methods you can use to increase blood circulation under the scalp:

- A good scalp massage every day. Place both hands on the sides of your head, close to the base of your scalp. Apply pressure to your scalp, with your fingertips, working in a circular motion. Continue this motion as you massage toward the front of your head. Reverse the movement going toward the back of your head. Place your fingertips on your scalp and massage in a back and forth motion across your head. Do this for two to fifteen minutes at a time.
- Lying on a slanted board, head down toward the ground (or with your head hanging off the edge of your bed) will increase the blood flow to the head. Do this for five to fifteen minutes, preferably first thing in the morning. Do not continue this practice if you are ill or feel nauseated.
- Thirty minutes of aerobic exercise at least three times a week. Just do it!

COSMETIC SOLUTIONS

For those folks who have suffered hair loss from any of the reasons described in this chapter, unless you have permanent damage that resulted in 100 percent baldness, there are some natural-hair-care solutions you may want to explore. Seek professional consultation as to what options are possible for your hair's needs. After years of dealing with so much damage, many braiders have become experts in styling and concealing hair loss.

Over the years I have learned many techniques from Master braiders across the country. Each technique is truly innovative, and as unique as its creator. One of my greatest joys has been creating Afrocentric styles for women of all ages who suffer with this situation. It's a great alternative to wearing a wig.

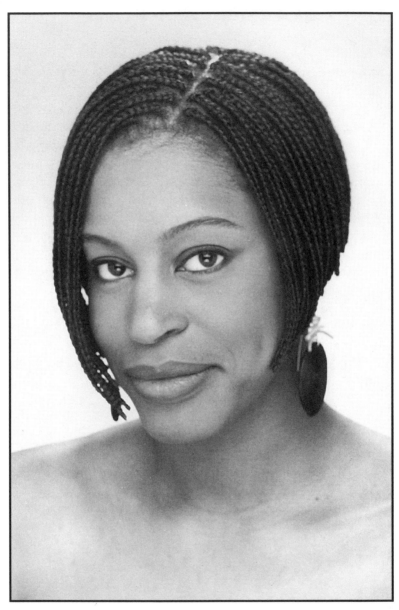

A single-braid bob style with synthetic hair is the best braided solution for Wendy's hair recovery. The weak edges were left untouched under the braids in the front, so as not to damage the area further with stress to the scalp.

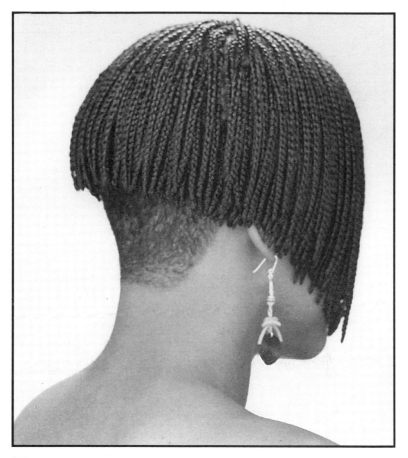

The lower back of her hair was cut close. It was too short and weak to try to grab for single braids. Above the cut, short single braids cascade down to complete the "bob" look. Wendy can shampoo and condition her hair once per week. She can even have deep steam treatments without the fear of her braids falling out. This style is inexpensive, and it will last two months. *(Stylist, Avion Julien)*

BRAIDS

If you have hair around your hairline and it is fairly strong, it can be used to create a foundation for a style that would conceal thin patches in the crown area of the head. Following are two popular techniques that use human hair to help create a full head of texturized hair to conceal alopecia areas.

BRAID WEAVE—INTERLOCK METHOD

This is a cornrow-based weave. The extension hair is cornrowed into the hair in a pattern that is best suited to conceal the alopecia area. One side of the extension hair is left out of the braid, and serves as an anchor to the other side of the extension. The side that is left out serves to conceal the cornrow braid as well. If the whole head is done, you would only see loose hair, which could then be cut and styled accordingly.

WEFTED WEAVING

This technique is not really applicable for serious cases of alopecia. The hair is cornrowed in a pattern to conceal the alopecia areas. Loose human hair that has been machine-stitched together to create what is called a weft is then sewn to these cornrows. The loose hair conceals the rows and the alopecia areas.

It's not what's on your head that counts, but how you feel about yourself. I am here to encourage you to express and celebrate the best of yourself through your natural beauty. Hopefully, with the information I've shared, you will be encouraged to make choices that enhance your well-being. Even if you decide chemical processing is for you, your choice can now be made with all the facts in hand. If you do decide to wear your hair in a natural style, Chapter Three provides crucial information on coming clean with your hair. Either way, you now have the tools at hand to develop a treatment plan for your hair, as well as feeling empowered to seek out products that will best nourish it and help minimize the degree of damage described in this chapter.

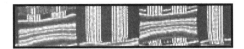

COMING CLEAN—SHAMPOO
AND GROOMING 101

T HE PURPOSE OF A SHAMPOO is to cleanse the hair and scalp of dust, dirt, grease, and oil. Unfortunately, shampooing also results in the loss of natural oils and moisture the hair needs. Conditioners were developed to replenish the hair's moisture content and its suppleness. In order to choose the most effective shampoo and conditioner for your hair, you must understand several things. The most important are: the pH factor, and whether your hair is dry, normal, or oily.

JUST THE pHACTS, MA'AM

The abbreviation pH stands for potential hydrogen. It describes the acidic and alkaline volume ratio in a shampoo. The ratio is measured on a number scale from 1 to 14. A pH-balanced shampoo usually describes a shampoo that is chemically balanced to clean your hair without stripping it of natural moisture and oil. It rates between 5 and 7 on the pH scale; 6.5 to 7 is pretty much the norm for pH-balanced shampoos.

I doubt you will ever actually see this listed, but just for your information, substances that are on either end of the pH scale—1 to 3 or 11 to 14—will definitely damage the skin and hair.

THE pH SCALE

From 1 to 5—acidic products:

Lemon rinses
Color rinses
Hydrogen peroxide (used in permanent coloring)
Neutralizers (for chemical straighteners)

From 5 to 9—alkaline products:

Soap shampoos (olive- or coconut-oil based)
Conditioners
Cream rinses
Antidandruff shampoos
Hair preparations: pomades, hair grease, petroleum, or beeswax-based products, etc.
Semipermanent color
Permanent color

From 10 to 14:

Chemical straighteners
Bleaches (superdestructive products)

SHAMPOOS

Most commercially manufactured shampoos are pH-balanced. The only exceptions are the highly alkaline clarifying shampoos. These shampoos are designed to remove buildup from hard water, gels, sprays, mousses, pool chemicals, etc. You don't need shampoos that have a lot of perfumes and other additives, so you shouldn't need a clarifying shampoo unless you have hard water. You also don't need a medicated shampoo unless you are under a dermatologist's care for a specific hair and scalp problem such as eczema or scalp lesions.

Also, stay away from protein and balsam shampoos. They do not clean the hair very well, and they weigh down the cuticle. Be wary of shampoos that have too much lather. Their alkaline content is very high, removing all the natural oils from your hair, leaving it dry and brittle. The best kinds of shampoos have oil bases, such as olive oil, jojoba oil, and coconut oils

WHY IS YOUR HAIR DRY, NORMAL, OR OILY?

Let's take a closer look at your hair. Is it normal, dry, or oily? Pop quiz! What gland is responsible for this condition? (I'm going to assume you paid close attention to the highlighted terms in Chapter One.) You're right! The sebaceous gland. The activity of this gland is directly responsible for creating a normal, dry, or oily environment on your scalp. What's normal is a relative state. What may be normal for your very curly hair is not normal for his wavy hair, or her straight hair. It's a good thing for very curly hair to be somewhat oily—not too much, not too little. Wavy or straight hair would not do well under the normal oil conditions of very curly hair.

Symptoms of Dry Hair
• Your hair is hard and brittle to the touch
• You have tiny flakes of dry skin from your scalp

• Whenever you comb your hair it sheds and/or you have hair breakage

Symptoms of Oily Hair
• Hair strands feel slick or greasy all the time
• Development of heavy flaking that will fall or can be scratched up from the scalp
• Pimples on the forehead close to the hair line

Normal Hair
• No flaking from the scalp
• No excessive oiliness
• No excessive dryness

All hair textures share a common problem. If the sebaceous gland is overly active, a dandruff condition results. An underactive gland would create a dandruff condition as well. As mentioned previously, the malfunctioning of this gland can happen as a result of age, diet, emotional stress, lack of exercise, drugs, chemical relaxers, hair dyes, and shampoos. During adolescence, oily skin and greasy hair are almost expected. And anyone who has been chemically straightening their hair over a period of time is sure to notice some type of scalp problem.

There is no absolute formula guaranteed to make the sebaceous gland work perfectly all of the time, but the closer you bring your hair and body back to their natural states, if the gland is not permanently damaged, the better the chance of improving the results. The body has incredible healing and rejuvenation powers. However, the hair cannot take care of itself. You will have to aid in this process.

The outer layer of the hair shaft is called the cuticle, which is made up of microscopic layers of scales that determine the hair's porosity level—what will or will not enter the hair shaft (remember, as we told you in Chapter One, the hair shaft and the follicle are the same; it is the follicle under the skin, and when it grows through the scalp and hardens it becomes the hair shaft). The ability to absorb any shampoo, conditioner, hair oil, chemical relaxer, or dye is determined by whether the scales that make up the cuticle are open or closed. If the scales are closed, then the absorption level is very low and nothing can enter the cuticle. Your hair will be described as having what is called low porosity. This condition could also account for dryness, and a brittle hair shaft. You will need to be careful in your choice of shampoos and conditioners. You will need a shampoo that is capable of opening the cuticle without being too strong for the follicle, and a conditioner that is deep penetrating but able to close the cuticle.

If the cuticle scales are wide open, your hair will be described as being very porous. The cuticle will absorb everything that is put on the hair. The absorption rate is very high, but the retention of moisture is very low. The hair is frayed, brittle and dry. In this situation the hair shaft is not able to retain any of the benefits of good products. One would have to shampoo and condition the hair frequently since the hair is not retaining any of the benefits of the product on a long-term basis. The products one would be using would be based on hair type. If the high porosity is due to chemical damage, you should only use the mildest of products, shampooing and conditioning the hair on a weekly basis, no heat, thermal curling, or hot temperature dryers, until the cuticle has regenerated itself. This could take about seven to nine weeks.

Your hair could be very porous due to genetics. A simple way to determine the porosity of your hair is:

Take a strand of your hair, stretch it out, and run your index finger and your thumb together up and down the shaft. If it feels rough then it's porous, the cuticles are open. If it feels very smooth, then the cuticle scales are closed and not porous.

SHAMPOO INGREDIENTS

There are many good natural-hair-care products on the market. Some are more effective than others, but that judgment is truly left up to the user.

I'm sure you know what does not work on your hair. Hopefully, we can shed some light on what will work. We are all trying to obtain the most natural products available for our bodies, but I must take time here to discuss the word *natural* as it applies to hair-care products.

In recent years, there have been major discussions in government agencies that approve "natural" products, from food substances to body-care products. My research for this book has brought a few more facts to my attention, and now I'm bringing them to you as clearly as I know how.

Almost every natural shampoo and conditioner I have come across has a foundation of chemical compounds that enhance whatever herbal, nutty, fruity, or oily natural extract that probably tops the list of ingredients on the bottle's label. I'm sorry, but no herbal tea, fruit juice, or nut oil is going to cleanse your hair without a mild detergent. (You can shut your mouth now.) What alarmed me was when I looked up these chemical substances on the label I saw the word *detergent*. All I could think of was washing clothes and floors. Well, according to Webster (yes, I had to go there), a detergent is a cleansing substance made from chemical compounds (meaning substances mixed together), rather than fats and—are you ready—lye!

Now refer back to the definition of pH balance. The detergent needed to cleanse our hair, that is present in most natural shampoos, is not necessarily a bad thing. These detergents combined with the oils of coconuts, olives, and palm nuts, serve as excellent cleansing agents. They are at the top of the list of ingredients on every shampoo that claims to be all natural. The same is true of a lot of conditioners. A lot of teas and oils will condition your hair. If your hair is natural, you follow a very good diet, take the appropriate supplements, have a stress-free environment, and you exercise at least three times a week, these totally natural ingredients might work for you.

The marketing dollars spent by some of the top "natural," "botanical," and "aroma therapeutic" companies add up to enough to feed and educate a small country. Just read the labels; you'll see what I mean. Their claim to fame is their whole botanical concept, and many of them get away with just listing the fruit, vegetable, tea and herbal content in the product without listing its chemical constituent.

The more reputable companies will list palm nuts, and also list cocamidopropylamine oxide beside it. This is a mild detergent, and has a good conditioning effect on the hair.

I will state for the record that there is nothing on the market that is promoted as all natural—that is truly all natural—that can also be effective on our hair given the chemical and thermal abuse, the environment, and the basic stress levels we live in from day to day. But many of the all natural conditioners on the market that combine mild chemical agents with herbs, fruit, healthy oil and vegetable extracts, can produce a positive benefit to even the most damaged hair.

There are some basic ingredients found in all good cleansing, moisturizing shampoos. Look for:

Sodium laureth sulfate: A mild, cleansing agent derived from coconut oil. It is used in many products for its excellent foaming and cleansing properties. It gently, yet very effectively, removes grease from the hair and skin.

Propylene glycole: Derived from coconut oil, it attracts and locks in moisture.

Lauramide DEA: Derived from palm trees, it is a gentle foam enhancer.

Cocamidopropylamine oxide: Extracted from palm nuts, it is a mild detergent with conditioning properties.

If you see these names among the ingredients listed on a shampoo bottle, it has the makings of a good shampoo for hair that needs moisture—which is most of our hair types.

SHAMPOO/CONDITIONER PRODUCTS

These products are designed for those who have to shampoo their hair frequently, and who don't have time to do a separate conditioning routine every time. The little bit of conditioner that is present in the shampoo will have to suffice until you are able to take the time to do it right. Additionally, always try to use a leave-in conditioner when forced to use these products over long periods of time.

CLARIFYING SHAMPOOS

Trying to shampoo your hair with hard water is very difficult. This water contains a lot of minerals—like copper, calcium, and iron, to name just a few. A shampoo that provides more than adequate suds with normal water conditions will barely make suds with hard water. If you find it very difficult for soap to lather, you probably have hard water.

If you live in an area with hard water, you must use this type of shampoo to remove mineral buildup from your hair. These minerals respond to the static electricity that our hair carries naturally. Hair carries a negative charge and water carries a positive charge. What is interesting is that the more damaged your hair is, the greater its negative charge. So damaged hair can't win for losing in that it will inadvertently attract more minerals from the water to itself. Over time the mineral buildup will make the hair very hard to manage, and affect any coloring process done to the hair.

Softening agents need to be added to the water, and a clarifying shampoo will have to be used, which is the last thing someone with damaged hair would want. Why? Because it will only dry out the damaged hair even more. But don't despair, because the good thing is that clarifying shampoos have a high alkaline content and so they swell up the hair shaft, causing the cuticle to become more porous and ready to receive a deep-conditioning treatment (DCT), which you should apply. (Leave the DCT in for the specified time and rinse really well. Next, do a lemon rinse, or the apple-cider-vinegar rinse, and apply a leave-in conditioner that has an excellent, light oil base, and everything should be just fine.)

MEDICATED SHAMPOOS

These shampoos are over-the-counter products for scalp and hair problems. The main active ingredient in a good dandruff shampoo is salicylic acid. This substance is found in many herbs, including cloves, peppermint, and yarrow. It has antibacterial properties. Mild flaking conditions are usually alleviated with the consistent use of these products over a short period of time. If these products are not arresting the problem, please seek medical attention.

THE RIGHT SHAMPOO FOR YOU

When thinking about whether your hair is normal, oily, or dry, the only condition that needs special consideration when choosing a shampoo is oily hair, so I've provided a separate set of instructions on the page to follow.

NORMAL AND DRY HAIR

Normal and dry hair need moisturizers. Dry hair needs more than normal, but in general "natural" shampoos will say "dry" or "dry and damaged" on the label. Look for the ingredients discussed earlier in this chapter when choosing your shampoo. Any other moisturizers combined with those ingredients will work fine to cleanse your hair without stripping it of its natural oils. You don't have to have an overprocessed head to use these products; it simply means they contain extra emollients (moisturizers). Shampoo once a week.

OILY HAIR

You want to minimize the constant, natural oil secretions that form on your hair shaft. Use a mild pH-balanced shampoo designed for oily hair. It should not have any additives, perfumes, etc. Follow shampoo with a cream rinse for detangling. After combing out and grooming your hair (twisting, braiding, setting, etc.), try to let it dry naturally. Heat activates your sebaceous glands, stimulating the flow of oil. Shampoo twice a week. Always follow with a cream rinse for detangling.

You need rinses that are of an acidic nature, but that also have conditoning properties, like lemon rinses, herbal teas (lavender, cypress, rosemary, birch), and apple cider vinegar.

CHEMICALLY DAMAGED HAIR

Hair that has been damaged due to chemical processing—whether from relaxers, dye, or over-processing—needs to be treated with the utmost care. The best shampoos to use are those that are for-mulated for dry and damaged hair. These products are designed to replenish the moisture to your hair. They are oil-based, and have humectants (substances that attract moisture). Try to use a condi-tioner made by the same manufacturer. They are usually designed to enhance each other's effectiveness. "Deep conditioning" are key words you should be looking for on the conditioner's label. If not present, go to another product line of similar quality. Don't expect to see immediate results. It usually takes a short time to damage hair, and a long time to rejuvenate it.

Be very gentle with your hair throughout the shampooing process.

- Wet the hair with warm water.
- Apply a small amount of shampoo (the size of a quarter) to the palm of your hand. This amount will usually cover a head

twenty-four inches in diameter, hair of short to medium length.
Use a little more shampoo for thicker or longer hair.
• Gently massage the hair and scalp with the balls of your finger-
tips.
• Rinse with a mild, even flow of warm water.
• Towel dry to remove excess water.
• Apply a deep conditioner, follow the manufacturer's instruc-
tions to the letter.
• Rinse the conditioner out very well. Any conditioner mistak-
enly left in the hair can cause further breakage.
• Try to air dry if you can.
• Follow this regimen once a week.

HOW TO SHAMPOO NATURAL HAIR

• Wet and saturate your hair with water.
• Apply shampoo to the scalp, hairlines (front and back), and to
the ends of the hair.
• Massage the scalp with your fingertips, moving from the front
to the back areas. Work the shampoo into the hair, gently
stretching it out as you go along.
• Let the water run through your hair to rinse out the shampoo,
then repeat the process (shampooing the hair twice is usually adequate unless the hair is excessively oily, then a third time would
be necessary). Make sure to rinse the hair thoroughly, letting the
water run through the hair until it runs clear (free of soap) in the
tub or sink.
• Take a towel and dry your hair to remove excess water, then
apply conditioner to the hair. Follow product instructions as to
length of time you should leave the conditioner on your hair.
After the designated waiting time, rinse the hair thoroughly.
Take the towel and squeeze the excess water out of your hair,
then separate into small sections to pat the scalp dry.

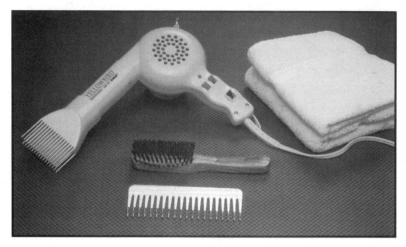

Preparations for shampooing natural hair; two large towels (one for draping over your shoulders and the other for drying your hair); a wide-toothed comb; and a blow dryer with a hair comb attachment.

CONDITIONERS

Conditioners are designed to replenish the moisture, body, strength, and manageability of the hair. In many cases, they replace the natural oils that have been washed away by the shampoo. The conditioner penetrates the cuticle, to be absorbed by the cortex, in an effort to repair any damage that may have been done to the strand. The conditioner falls in the acidic realm of the pH scale, between 3 and 5. Whatever is

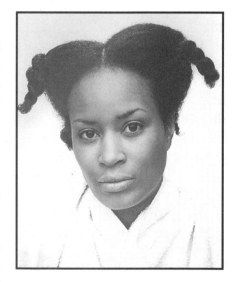

Part your hair into sections and double-twist each section. Hold the hair in one of the sections close to the base of the scalp.

not absorbed by the cuticle gets rinsed away, and the cuticle is closed by the water used to rinse—and the acidic nature of the conditioner.

Deep conditioners are best for normal, dry, and damaged hair. If you're using a heat-derived styling method, you must also apply moisturizing oil, or a leave-in conditioner.

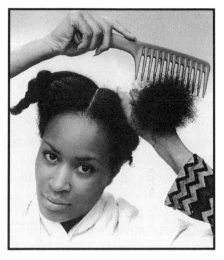

CONDITIONING INGREDIENTS TO LOOK FOR

The following ingredients are safe, effective conditioning agents to use on any hair type. Always read the label before buying any shampoo or conditioner.

Take the comb while holding the hair close to the base of the scalp and comb out the ends very gently, using short strokes. After clearing the top, take the comb down to the base of the section, comb gently in an upward motion, bringing the comb through the hair from the base of the scalp to the ends of the hair. As each section is combed out, twist the hair loosely back and clip to prepare for drying the hair.

Cetheth 20: Moisturizer derived from palm oil
Panthenol: Moisturizer and conditioning agent derived from vitamin B_5
Cetearyl alcohol: Moisturizer and thickening agent

LEAVE-IN CONDITIONERS

These are very acidic and rich in emollients. They are generally used if you are blow-drying or thermal curling the hair. They provide moisture to the hair shaft and then close the cuticle, providing a protective coating ready for any heat-based styling procedure.

NATURAL CONDITIONERS

Many of the active ingredients found in the best conditioners come from an organic source, mother nature. Quite a few of them can be found in your kitchen. Herbal teas can be made into wonderful rinses that are anti-bacterial, penetrate and strengthen the cortex, stimulate the scalp for improved blood circulation, and improve hair growth. Fruit and vegetable pulps can replenish the moisture and oils that are constantly robbed from our hair on a daily basis.

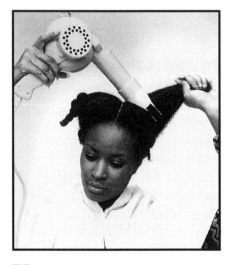

Fruit conditioners can be blended into a paste and applied to the hair. Do not let the mixtures sit around for a long period of time. Once the skin of the fruit or vegetable is pierced the active ingredients are ready to start working for you. Once they are applied to the hair, put on a plastic cap and leave it on for twenty to thirty minutes. Rinse well under warm water.

Untwist a section and hold the hair at the base of the scalp and take the blow dryer (set the temperature on the warm setting) and comb through the ends gently, using an upward stroke. Continue combing upward while stretching out the hair.

These types of conditioning treatments are not recommended to loc wearers who twist their locs down to the scalp.

Try these:

• *Avocado:* The oil and pulp are rich in potassium, sulfur, and vitamins A, B, and E. It is an excellent conditioner for the hair as well as the skin. It replenishes the oils and coats the cuticle, leaving the hair feeling smooth and soft.

• *Banana:* The pulp is a great biodegradable moisturizer and lubricant, excellent for dry hair. It is a wonderful humectant, locking in moisture and coating the hair shaft, leaving the hair smooth. The pulp is rich in potassium and vitamins A, B, and C.

• *Seaweed and Lecithin:* Seaweed is rich in iodine, amino acids, mineral salts, and vitamins A, B, C, and E. It is a softening and conditioning agent, and has anti-bacterial properties. Lecithin is an emollient and a natural emulsifier. It serves to seal the nourishing elements of any seaweed mixture into the cuticle.

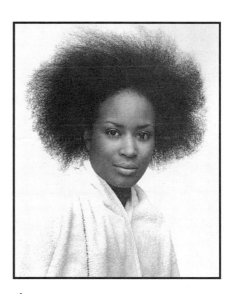

After each section is combed out, part the hair and massage a small amount of moisturizing hair oil into the scalp. The hair is now ready to be styled.

There are many different types of seaweeds. To make things easy, I would suggest you use an extract or a powder like Agar-Agar. Both Agar-Agar and lecithin can be easily found in any health food store.

Both of these products must be mixed with tepid water and will congeal if the right consistency is not achieved. It should be on the thick syrupy side. Use immediately.

CREAM RINSES

These products are designed to smooth the cuticle and detangle the hair. They make the hair more manageable, and they are excellent for use on children's hair (no pain!).

DEEP CONDITIONERS/RECONSTRUCTIVE CONDITIONERS

These conditioners are protein based, and are designed to penetrate the cuticle and alter the cellular structure of the cortex. This action replenishes moisture and repairs damage done to the follicle. Some deep conditioners infuse vitamins into the cuticle and further nourish the cortex.

These products are almost always activated by heat, to aid in opening the cuticle. They are left on the hair an average of twenty minutes, and they must be thoroughly washed out. If traces are left undetected, they will continue working, and cause breakage of the hair shaft.

Reconstructors are very heavy, batterlike mixtures. They are made of proteins, fatty acids, and other chemical constituents that retain moisture and seek to repair damage done to the cortex. As a rule they don't require heat. They just need time to work, and are usually left in about thirty minutes. They must also be washed out very well.

Beware of deep conditioners that have mineral and/or petroleum oils listed as part of their ingredients. Using this type of conditioner after you shampoo your hair defeats the purpose. You would have to shampoo your hair about four to five times to remove the heavy-duty coating of oil left on the hair shaft. Nothing can penetrate the cuticle with this type of coating, and with continued use you will develop a scalp problem. Your pores will be clogged, and the sebaceous gland will not be able to produce the sebum it needs to lubricate your scalp naturally. It doesn't matter if your hair is natural or chemically straightened, light oil bases, such as almond, olive, avocado, or calendula are best for your hair.

HOT OIL TREATMENTS

Hot oil conditioning formulas, when heat activated (heating cap or steam machine), penetrate the cuticle and go into the cortex to strengthen and lubricate the hair shaft. They usually have an ingredient of an acidic nature, that when rinsed out will serve to close the cuticle. The oil will then lightly coat the hair strand, to lock in moisture and protect the cuticle.

HAIR PREPARATIONS

This is the professional term for grease, pomades, and oils for the hair. Pomades and grease are definitely not what you need to put in your hair for health and manageability. Generally, these products are petroleum based or beeswax based. They will not get rid of dryness. On the contrary, they will create a situation where your hair will not be able to absorb any of the conditioning agents it needs. What these products do is coat the hair shaft so the cuticle cannot open. No matter what type of shampoo is used, it will not cleanse the hair with the average two to three wash cycles. You will be there for a long time, and in most cases you will not be able to remove the heavy, petroleum-based or mineral-based products from your hair. When the cuticle cannot open, the natural oils from the sebaceous gland cannot be released. A dry scalp will develop. It will also set the stage for other problems.

OILS THAT CAN BE APPLIED TO THE SCALP

Rosemary oil: Stimulates growth, has antiseptic properties, good for dandruff, excellent for giving shine to dark hair
Sage oil: Astringent, stimulates growth, kills bacteria; it is said to have the ability to darken graying hair
Jojoba oil: Smooths and conditions curly hair, good for a dry scalp

Sweet almond oil: Contains vitamins E and F, good for an itchy scalp, mild and easily absorbed
Avocado oil: Rich in potassium and sulfur, vitamins A, D, and E, easily absorbed
Evening primrose oil: Moisturizes and conditions the hair
Calendula oil: Moisturizes, very good in soothing scalp and skin conditions like eczema.

HOW TO APPLY OILS TO THE SCALP

• Rub a small amount of the product onto the back of your hand. If it absorbs easily, quickly, and feels good, then you would probably want to put it in your hair.
• Part the hair into four sections, then subdivide each section into two, then four, then eight sections. Each will end up about an inch apart. Apply the product sparingly all over the head.
• Take this opportunity to give yourself a good scalp massage.
• Apply the oil every day for four days, take a break for two days, and at the end of that second day examine your hair and scalp. If hair is retaining oil, but not overly so, continue this regimen. If it is too oily, cut down to once a week.

DRYING YOUR HAIR

There are three effective ways to dry your natural hair.

AIR DRYING

After shampooing, towel-dry your hair. If you have a short natural style, then there is nothing else to do except oil it. If your hair is more than three inches long, separate hair into small sections. Oil the scalp, if necessary.

HOOD DRYING

Towel-dry the hair after shampooing. Oil the scalp lightly, if you need to. Section the hair in as many parts as you need to make it manageable. Twist the sections in two-stranded twists and sit under the hood dryer on a low setting until your hair is dry (approximately twenty to thirty minutes).

BLOW DRYING

Use a 1,200-watt blow dryer with a comb attachment. Towel-dry the hair after shampooing, conditioning, and applying a leave-in conditioner. Take a wide-toothed comb, make your appropriate sections, and hold the blow dryer on a low temperature in one hand and your section of hair with the other hand. Put the comb of the blow dryer at the base of the section of hair, then pull through the section gently and slowly. Continue the process until you have completed the entire head.

NO PAINS, NO STRAINS FOR NATURAL MANES: HOW TO COMB OUT NATURAL HAIR

WET AND DRY

If your hair is more than two inches long, try to part it into small sections (about four square inches each). Hold the hair at the base of the scalp, take a wide-toothed comb, and, starting at the ends of the hair, comb through gently, working your way down to the base of the head. Make sure to include a detangling conditioner/rinse in your hair-care regimen.

SCALP DISORDERS

Very often scalp disorders are neglected and turn into serious problems, that could have been avoided if immediate action was first taken to alleviate the problem. The hair and scalp serve as an indicator as to what is going on in the body. A scalp disorder will either come from an internal or external problem. In either case seek professional help from a dermatologist.

When in doubt, check it out!

DANDRUFF

When left untreated a serious dandruff ailment can result in itching that will lead to infections, scabbing, swelling, redness of the scalp, and temporary or permanent hair loss. Dandruff is highly contagious since bacteria and fungus are present in this scalp disorder. Combs and brushes must not be shared by family members. The person with the disorder should sterilize their combs and brushes as well. After a successful treatment you don't want to re-infect your scalp all over again.

This condition may be due to:

- malfunctioning of the sebaceous gland
- dry scalp
- scalp irritation due to the use of harsh chemicals (relaxers, dyes, etc.)
- improper diet (starchy and fatty foods)
- poor circulation
- lack of personal hygiene
- stress, nervousness, and anxiety

There are two types of dandruff:

- Pityriasis Steatoides (oily dandruff)
  This is a very serious form of dandruff. It is characterized by

large, yellowish scales. It mixes with the sebum, causing it to stick to the hair and scalp. This type of dandruff cannot be scratched up or easily removed, and the scalp is often infected and inflamed.

- Pityriasis Capitis Simplex (dry dandruff)
  This dandruff is characterized by small white powdery scales and an itchy scalp. These flakes easily dislodge themselves from the scalp. How much time has passed from its inception will determine whether or not a regimen of regular hair brushing, and shampooing with a medicated shampoo, will arrest the flaking.

The body naturally sheds dead skin every thirty days. It is usually invisible due to daily bathing and rubbing of one's skin on a regular basis. The shedding increases considerably when one has a serious case of dandruff. I cannot stress the importance of seeking medical attention from a dermatologist to diagnose as well as provide the proper medication to treat the problem.

In cases that are not as serious as those mentioned above, here are some methods you can try to arrest your problem:

- Treat your hair and scalp with great care. Comb and brush up the flakes, being careful not scratch, puncture, or irritate the scalp.
- Shampoo your hair twice, leaving the second shampoo lather on the scalp and hair for seven minutes before rinsing with warm water.
- Shampoo your hair two times per week. Use medicated over-the-counter shampoos. Look for products that contain salicylic acid and sulfur as active ingredients. They are very effective in peeling the surface layers of the scalp and removing dandruff scales.
- Rinse your hair with an anti-dandruff rinse. Towel dry and apply anti-dandruff oil to the scalp with a cotton ball.
- Change the brand of medicated shampoo if you see the shampoo is not working. After constant use, sometimes hair will de-

velop a resistance to a particular shampoo's formation of active ingredients.

• Give yourself two weeks to follow this treatment plan. If there is no change, seek medical attention.

TINEA (RINGWORM)

This is a fungus that appears on the scalp as white or red patches. It is highly contagious. There is hair loss around the infected area. This infection can also appear on the skin. It requires immediate medical attention.

SEBORRHEA

This appears as an unusual amount of oil on the hair. It produces scales that are much thicker than the ones found in the scalp for oily dandruff. Under these scales the scalp is infected by inflamed oil glands. This inflammation is caused by overstimulation and secretion from the sebaceous glands.

SOOTHING ANTIDANDRUFF RINSE AND OIL

Rinse

Take five tablespoons of each of these fresh or dried herbs

• Birch
• Rosemary
• Eucalyptus

Pour four cups of water into a glass pot with the herbs. Boil for twenty minutes. Cover the pot and let it cool. Strain the herbs and use the tea for the rinse.

Oil

This soothing oil uses the same herbal ingredients and quantities. Place herbs in a glass canning jar and add eight ounces of almond oil. Leave this mixture in a cool place for two weeks, then strain the herbs, and use oil as described earlier in this chapter.

DIET FOR HEALTHY HAIR

You may be wondering what your diet has to do with your hair? Everything! When you come to our salon for the first time, we have a consultation. You fill out a questionnaire, which tells us about your hair and your dietary habits. If your hair is dry, brittle, and falling out, and you eat a lot of red meat, drink at least four cups of coffee a day, and you don't drink any water, well, that's half of the problem—and the beginnings of the solution—right there.

The stress that comes with the caffeine in coffee directly affects the nervous system, which in turn goes straight to the papilla. Your nerves will run your hair out real fast! The red meat with no veggies, and lack of H_2O, is not only a prescription for baldness, but also to a whole host of other diseases due to improper elimination. You are what you eat. No product you can buy in the store will ever be able to make you have better hair without first making changes from within.

FOODS THAT HELP PROMOTE HEALTHIER HAIR

- Green, leafy vegetables (kale, spinach, collard, Swiss chard, dandelion)
- Asparagus
- Cabbage
- Carrots
- Cucumbers
- Tomatoes
- Whole grains, rice, pasta
- Beans (navy, red, adzuki, black-eyed peas, lentils)
- Fish
- Soy protein

- Chicken
- Raw Nuts and seeds

REMEMBER ♦ ♦ ♦

- Plenty of fruit (in season) will help curb cravings for sugar, which is a telltale sign of nutritional starvation.
- The body needs at least fifteen minutes of cardiovascular exercise every day.
- Practice deep-breathing exercises. The less stressed out you are, the less stressed your hair is.

I recommend establishing a relationship with a medical/holistic practitioner who will do a full physical, and determine what your body is lacking in the way of vitamins. Only blood work will tell you what you need to know to make decisions about taking the proper supplements. Improper supplementation can lead to a toxic situation. This body is God's finest creation. Study what works for you nutritionally. Take some courses, learn how to prepare healthy food. Watch your caloric intake. There is a lot of information available. "Seek and ye shall find."

Most of all, take your time. Organize yourself. Have quiet meditation and time for prayer every day. Commit to being good to yourself. Resolve to take care of yourself. Pay attention to your spirit, and you'll be on the path to regal movement in natural hair care, No Lye!

CHAPTER

FOUR

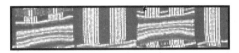

THE ART OF
BRAIDING

WHAT WE ARE EXPERIENCING in modern-day African-American culture is a celebration of a standard of beauty that is over 4,000 years old, grounded in traditional African art and religion.

THE ANCESTRAL LINK

THE HEAD HAS ALWAYS BEEN A SACRED PLACE

The concept of an extension is rooted in a spiritual, artistic, creative expression. The natural hair was extended in the form of a single braid, loc, wig, or three-dimensional hair sculpture through the use of various fibers from plants, animals, and tree bark. These fibers helped create elaborate hair adornments for rituals and ceremonies, or were worn as daily regalia according to one's status in the community.

Hairstyles were created for children as well as adolescent women and men. In southwest Africa, young Mabalantu women between the ages of sixteen and twenty participated in an initiation ceremony in which they wore extension braids that touched the ground.

The Massai warriors braided their hair throughout their teenage years. The hair grew down their backs, then as part of a rite of passage ceremony, they cut it off when they were ready to assume adult responsibilities in their community.

Khemetians (ancient Egyptians) showed their powerful status by shaving their heads and wearing wigs scented with essential oils. These wigs were dyed various colors, curled, twisted, and stiffened with beeswax.

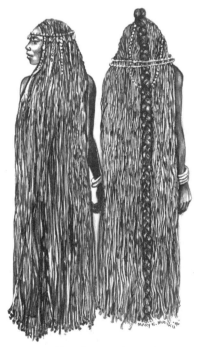

Young Mabalantu women wearing their traditional initiation hairstyle. *(Illustration by Mary E. Mudiku)*

Nigerians thread-wrapped elaborate hair sculptures, and devotees of the traditional Orisa (or-ee-sha) religion wore hairstyles depicting the energy of the deity Sango (pronounced shon-GO).

The use of dyes and mud was the only procedure even closely related to altering the state of one's natural hair. The intention was to change the color, never the texture.

BRIEF HISTORICAL "HAIR"-ITAGE

The art of braiding became very popular during the sixties, at the height of the civil rights and Black Power movements. The political and cultural expressions of African Americans became very focused, outspoken, and visible during this era. In fact, everyone from the hippies to the Panthers had long, natural hair. Visual statements about being natural were made, and people were proud of it.

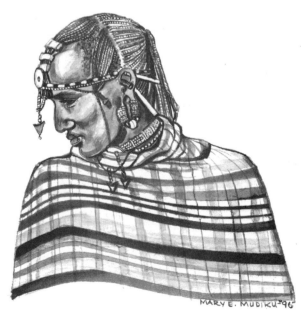

Traditional hairstyle of young Masai warrior. *(Illustration by Mary E. Mudiku)*

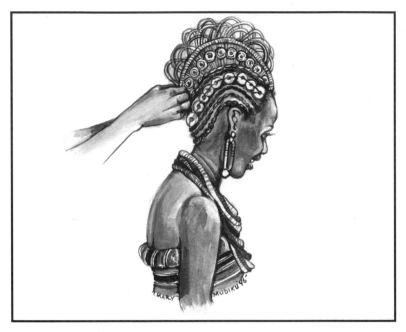

Young woman wearing traditional Yoruba Sango hairstyle. *(Illustration by Mary E. Mudiko)*

It spoke to an awakening of awareness as to what was morally and naturally correct treatment of one human being by another. Black women and men were coming into the consciousness of an African aesthetic. The "Afro" and braids were the ground-level introduction to natural hair care. Popular performing artists such as Cicely Tyson, Miriam Makeba, Stevie Wonder, and Roberta Flack were instrumental in carrying the natural imagery to an international level.

Throughout the seventies the art of braiding evolved from having your hair braided by a friend into a cottage industry for many African-American women and men. By the mid-eighties, anyone who was having their hair braided on a consistent basis in New York, Philadelphia, L.A., or D.C. carried a braider's signature on their heads. There was a distinct difference between East Coast and West Coast artistic expressions of the art form, very much akin to the analogies of jazz or hip hop music, and East Coast versus West Coast sound (no exclusion of St. Louis intended!).

The East Coast braiders were performing hairstyles with extensions and natural hair. Nationally, the initial extension-braiding work was large in size, and the point where the extension hair was added to the natural hair was very noticeable. There was a knot at the beginning of the braid. The West Coast braiders were innovators in that they began to make the braids smaller, and they refined the extension technique so the knots were no longer visible. Paving the way of this West Coast movement was Oakland, California's master sculptor, Malakia Hilton.

Malakia's work became evidence of the ancestral channeling that ushered in the appearance of a true crowning of our heads, and an awakening of our spirits to the ceremonial and regal sculptures that were performed only by hair sculptors of priestly stature. Their work was worn by high-ranking officials, other priests, and the kings and queens of ancient African cultures. Malakia unleashed this creative ancestral energy on Stevie Wonder's head, as his personal stylist during the mid-seventies and eighties. By creating Stevie Wonder's braids and beaded hair sculptures, Cicely Tyson's microbraids, and servicing anyone who desired this regal movement, she turned up the heat on the creative process of the art form. Through her influence, the big parts that exposed the scalp disappeared, knots in the extensions disappeared, and the use of semiprecious stones, fourteen-karat gold beads, gemstones, glass beads, and the incorporation of traditional hair wrapping within these hair sculptures became the norm.

When she moved from Oakland to Los Angeles, Malakia taught the art form at a local community center. Several of her students, including Margo, Sherifu, and Angela, moved to the East Coast. Once there, they influenced the style of Washington, D.C., braiders. Sherifu and Angela arrived in D.C. as students at Howard University. They began braiding to supplement their income as students. Margo also went to D.C., and soon thereafter Vernard Grey, owner of the Miya Art Gallery, asked her to braid in the gallery's window. Thus the process became performance art as well as a commercial enterprise. Miya Gallery became the first braiding salon in Washington, D.C.

Nawili Ayo, one of Malakia's most innovative students, arrived in D.C. in the late seventies, in response to an invitation by Mudiwa Bolong, a student of Sherifu and Angela. Nawili brought with her the next level of refinement to the art form. Her braiding technique was smaller than anything that had been done up to that time. The size of the braids had become what we know now as "microbraids."

At this size, the beadwork took on a life of its own. The work was the very essence of grace, opulence, and elegance with a depth that was yet a deeper expression of regal movement. The sculptures flowed liked water.

You were mesmerized by the way the different colors of the bead combinations wove an intricate tapestry of life on the head. Nawili taught her technique to five women: Anana, Fana, Kimako, Kecheku, and me. Fana traveled to D.C. with Nawili and remained there for many years, opening a salon and becoming a barber. Fana's adeptness with her new tools took her into creating hair sculptures that were trimmed or shaven very close to the scalp in one area, traditionally wrapped in another, and braided with bead-work in yet another. Fana's commitment to the art form led her to produce annual natural hair sculpture shows with fiber artist Januwa Moja. The shows grew to be a community artistic event, showcasing the work of local and international hair sculptors and fashion designers.

By the mid-eighties braiding had become very popular, but it was not an acceptable hairstyle for the corporate world. However, it was not long before braiding presented itself at the corporate world's doors demanding respect and recognition. The Marriott Hotel Corporation was sued by Washington, D.C., employee Cheryl Tatum. She was fired for wearing braids to work. With help from her stylist, Master Hair Sculptor Pamela Ferrell, Ms. Ferrell's husband Talib Din-Uqdah (owners of Cornrows & Company braiding salon), and Jesse Jackson, Ms. Tatum won the battle and set a great precedent. It is now against the law to discriminate against

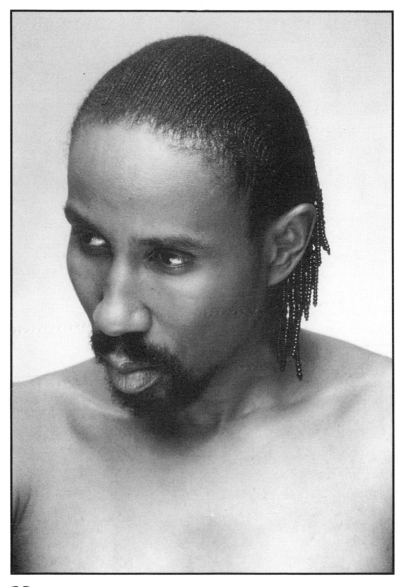

Micro cornrow extensions with black glass beads. Stanley Kinard wears an example of a West Coast cornrow style. The cornrows are braided very close together so that the scalp is not visible. *(Stylist, Tulani Kinard)*

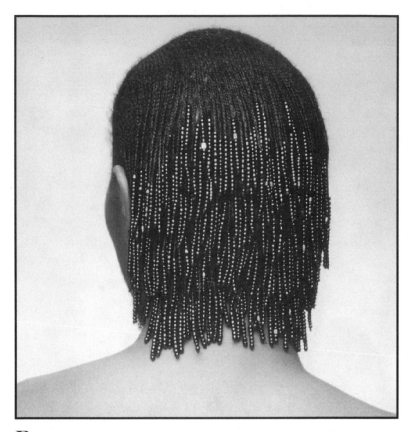

Back view of micro cornrows with extensions shows layers of single braids and beads that will last up to three months. The weight of the small glass beads on each braid helps to stimulate hair growth gently. The style can be washed and conditioned on a weekly basis. *(Stylist, Tulani Kinard)*

a person in a work environment because of his or her hair. In the words of one of our great ancestors, Frederick Douglass, "Power concedes nothing without a demand, never has and never will."

Our people fought to define our own aesthetic in the realm of natural hair care and won! The victory was sweet, and its sound traveled across this country. But the struggle continues.

Efforts are being made by trade organizations as well as braiding activists to create legislation and licenses for natural-hair-care professionals. To date, only New York (natural hair care) and Washington, D.C., (braiding) have such licenses.

NATURAL HAIR

Braiding your natural hair can be a wonderful, beautiful experience. I've included in the book some of the most attractive and easily worn hair "fashions" that have ever been created.

These styles can last up to two months, depending on the size of the braids. As a rule, any style that is braided in the medium to small size or smaller will last longer than larger-sized braids. These hairstyles may be washed and conditioned, but superemollient (moisturizing) shampoos and conditioners that are best for our hair will cause the braids to expand, loosen, and possibly fall off.

If you are wearing a cornrow style that is well braided and fairly small in size, and you are armed with a soft brush, light hair oils, gel, and a cotton scarf, your style will last several months.

Natural, individual braids and twists last a long time with the proper grooming. These may be washed and conditioned on a weekly basis.

There are styling options such as Bantu knots to break up any boredom with hanging braids or twists, as well as rolling the twists or braids on rods and changing the shape and look.

Natural styles are great for small children. Braids or twists can be sculpted in such a way that a new hairstyle can be created for them every week. The same methodology can also be applied to adults.

Mastering the technique of working with short, natural hair to create beautiful beaded hair sculptures was my impetus for learning how to braid. My mentor, Nawili Ayo, developed her technique of small braids without the use of extension fibers. The allure and brilliance of her work was obvious through her choice of semiprecious stones and crystals, along with African traditional wrapping techniques adapted to the use of nontraditional fibers. Her

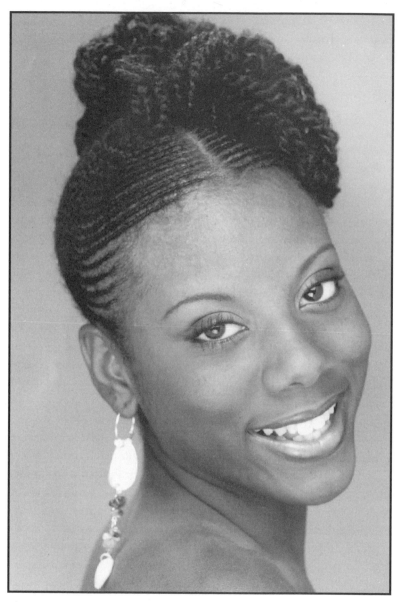

Arlene is wearing natural cornrows.

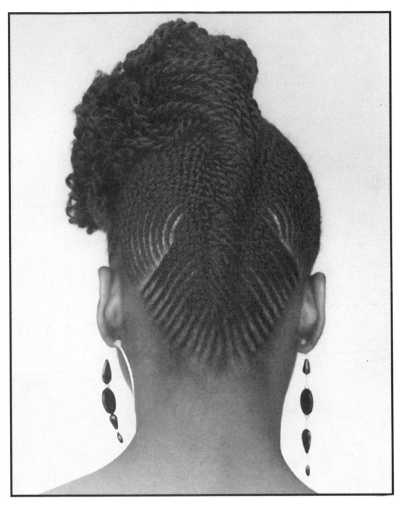

The ends are rolled from the back, resolving into an asymmetrical curly bun at the front of the model's head. This style will last two months. Biweekly grooming and sleeping with a silk scarf on every night will assure its beauty until the end. *(Stylist, Nicole James)*

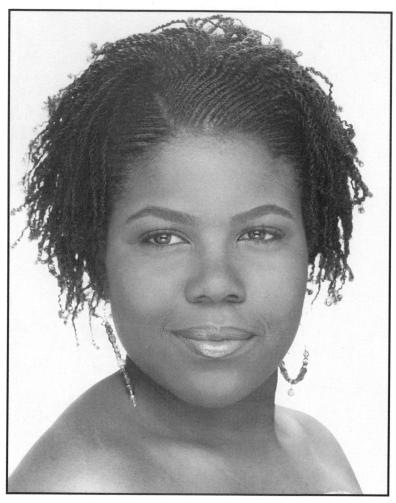

Talliah is wearing a combination style of natural micro cornrows on the front of her head with twists in the back. *(Stylist, Avion Julien)*

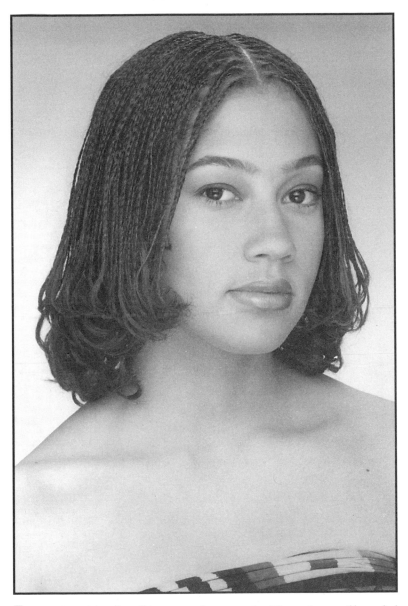

Imani's natural braids will last up to three months. The ends are softly curled under. Weekly shampooing and conditioning will keep her style looking great. *(Stylist, Avion Julien)*

expertise in any aspect of braiding was well known around the country, but her passion was for creating styles without the use of extensions. As a student, I observed the most damaged heads of hair transformed into works of art. The whole persona of a woman would change as she was totally empowered by the work done on her head. As I watched them get up from the floor their movement became poetic, each gesture of the hand, positioning of the body, the head. I witnessed regal movement over and over again. One of the most profound moments in my life was the first time I helped create this spirit within a woman.

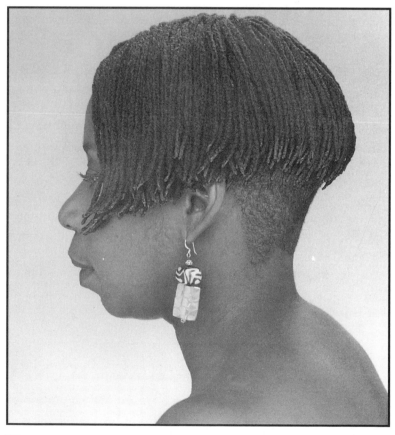

The nape of Iyanla's neck is faded to create a dramatic bob style.

Having your natural hair braided with ornamentation such as small beads or a thread wrap at the end of your cornrows will serve to stimulate your blood circulation, and the sebaceous glands in your scalp. The weight of small beads and the tension of the wrap serve as a daily scalp massage. They relax the scalp over a short period of time, enabling the follicle to emerge from the scalp, and the hair shaft to be in a healthier condition.

Each method, extensions or natural braiding, has its benefits. If you need a low-maintenance style to last three months, choose individual, extension braids.

EXTENSION BRAIDS

Extensions are used primarily for convenience. They hold your natural hair in place, and serve to protect it from daily exposure to the elements as well as wear and tear. Extensions also enable a hairstyle to last longer than styles using only natural hair; they're very durable. Some of the most popular looks and the fibers used to create them are:

STYLE	FIBER
Nu Locs	Yarn
Silky Locs	Synthetic hair
Genie Locs	Yarn
Extension locs	Yarn, Human hair
Individual braids	Human/Synthetic hair, Yarn
Cornrows	Human/Synthetic hair
Cornrows w/Individual braids	Human/Synthetic hair, Yarn
Braid weaves	Human hair
Thread wrapping	Cotton thread

Any of these styles can last up to three months *depending on the size of the braids or locs*. The extension fiber is added to the natural hair to give it support. It will keep the natural hair from fraying, slipping, or expanding inside the braid. Due to this kind of support, if

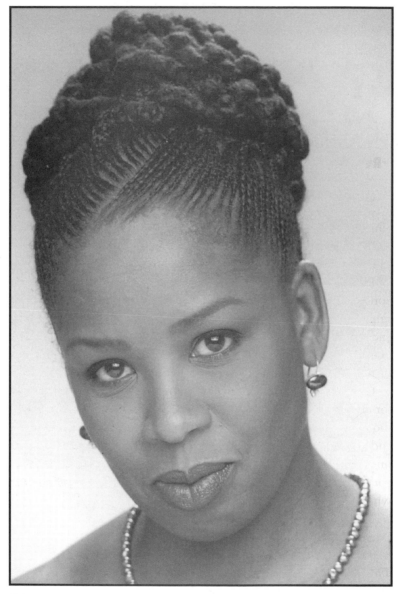

Esmerelda exudes the class and sophistication that only a skillfully executed cornrow hairstyle can create. Not too much, but always just enough, is the design that works best for business and personal affairs. This style is a combination of natural cornrows and acrylic yarn extensions.

the braids are designed to last three months, the hair can be washed and conditioned on a weekly basis without the threat of the style falling apart. When braided correctly, there is no damage to the hairline or scalp. Correct braiding also means there should be no pain during the process, or throughout the duration of the hairstyle.

PROS AND CONS OF DIFFERENT FIBERS

SYNTHETIC HAIR

This is loose hair braided together in a package.

It can be used for any braid style and Silky Locs.

Price: $2.99 to $5.99 per package.

Pros: Great for cornrows and individual braids. It is easy to wash, condition, and dry. There is no expansion of the braid. It can be singed, plus texturized with hot water, electric or thermal curling, and crimping irons. Look for the brand name Kanekelon. This brand is preferable if you want successful results when applying any of the finishing techniques that complete the hairstyle.

Cons: If braided too tightly, it will not "give." Don't try to wait for the pain to go away; take the braids out immediately. If you wait too long, you could cause traction baldness. If your skin is sensitive and you get rashes fairly easily, consider testing the fiber. Put on one braid and wear it overnight. Let it touch your skin; this gives you the chance to check for adverse reactions before braiding your whole head.

SYNTHETIC WEFTED HAIR

This is loose hair sewn together on a weft; it is used for track weaving.

Price: $12.00 to $20.00 per package.

Pros: It's fairly inexpensive compared to human hair. The texture lends itself to that of a "press and curl" of medium- to coarse-textured hair. If the fiber used is Kane Kelon, it can be curled with thermal implements.

Cons: It is not as easy to care for as human hair. It becomes stiff and unmanageable with age (after three to four weeks). Those with sensitive skin cannot use this fiber.

HUMAN HAIR

Pros: There are many different types and textures of human hair. If the hair is purchased from a reputable manufacturer (you can purchase a much cheaper quality of hair from a vendor, but I know your results will not be the same), you are able to get lengths varying from nine inches up to twenty-two inches. The color possibilities are endless. Hair can be mixed and blended to your exact specifications. It should be tangle free if handled properly, and the dyes used to attain the vast selection of colors should not bleed when the hair is wet.

Cons: The individual-braids style is not as durable with this fiber. You cannot wash the hair as often, and you cannot apply conditioners or shampoos that are *super*emollient. They will soften the hair, cause braid expansion, and the extension hair will begin to slide from the base and fray. This is also true of cornrow hairstyles using human hair as the extension. When shampooed, the cornrows will swell and your natural hair will curl inside and outside of the braid stitch.

This is not to say that this fiber cannot be used for individual (box) braids. However, be careful and make sure to have your hair done by an experienced braider whose work you admire.

OTHER TYPES OF EXTENSION HAIR

The following approximate price quotes are for manufactured hair weight, not for natural-hair-care professional services.

WET AND WAVY

This hair can be straightened with a blow dryer, set on rollers, thermal curled, or just wet with water and it will form a loose wave pattern. It comes loose and it can be sewn by hand or a machine to create a weft (thread band) to be used for track weaving. Loose, it can be used for braid weaves or individual braid hairstyles.

Price: ¼ pound costs $45.00. You would need approximately ½ pound of hair ($80.00) for an average-sized head of medium or small, shoulder-length individual braids. (This price does not include custom color hair blending.)

KINKY HAIR

Used in the extension loc, this hair is a blend of relaxed human hair and yak hair. It looks like an "Afro puff."

Price: ¼ pound costs $65.00. Hair for an average-sized head of medium individual locs in a bob style (short chin length) could easily cost $300.00.

RELAXED HAIR

This is used in wefted weaves or braid weaves. It is processed to look like straight, relaxed hair. It is loose hair, and can be sewn on a weft by hand or a machine to be used in tracking weaving. It can be roller set, thermal curled, or crimped.

Price: ¼ pound costs approx. $65.00.

YAK HAIR

This hair is very coarse and heavy, and comes from an animal called the yak. It is often blended with human hair to give it a softer texture. Used for track weaving and braid weaves, it can be roller set, thermal crimped, and curled.

Price: ¼ pound costs $50.00 to $60.00.

ACRYLIC YARN

This fiber is used for braids, twists, and wraps.

Price: $2.99 (small) to $5.99 (large) per skein, depending on the weight. One large skein could complete an average-sized head of shoulder-length, individual braids.

Pros: It is durable, lightweight, easy to wash, and quick to dry. It can be burned and dyed (the color cannot be lightened), and the older it gets the more it looks like locs.

Cons: The older acrylic yarn gets the better it looks, so folks tend to leave it in too long and risk losing the equity (hair growth) on their investment. It only comes in two colors: black and brown.

LAINE YARN

This is a wool fiber that is manufactured in France. Used for Senegalase twists, corkscrews, flat twists, and braids.

Price: It comes in skeins, which cost from $25.00 to $45.00 per skein. One large skein will complete an average-sized head of medium individual twists to the shoulders. It comes in black, dark brown, and light brown.

Pros: It is soft.

Cons: It is very porous. When wet, it takes a very long time to dry.

BRAIDING WITH EXTENSIONS: WHEN YOU (OR A FRIEND) WANT TO DO IT YOURSELF

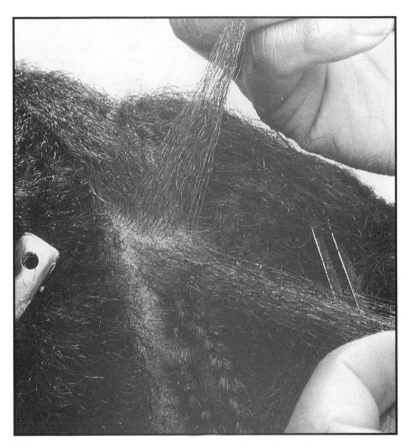

Part the hair into four large sections. Secure three of the sections by twisting or braiding them together and then part these sections into diagonal rows. Make smaller parts within these diagonal rows, then split each smaller section in half.

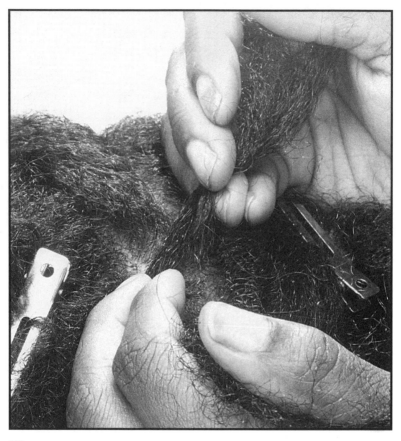

Take an amount of extension hair equal to the hair in the newly parted section of the diagonal row.

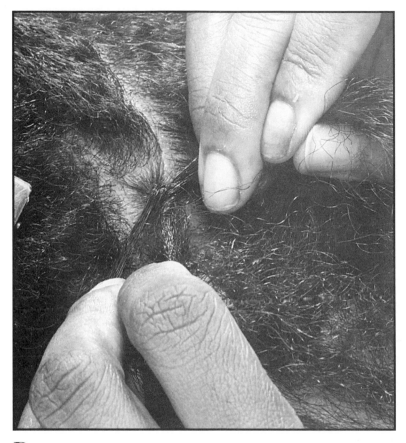

Divide the extension hair into these sections and attach/braid the extension hair into the natural hair.

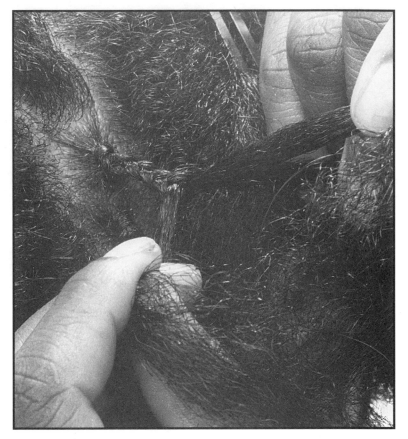

Continue braiding down, with the extension firmly anchored at the base of the scalp. Be careful not to pull the hair too tightly. It creates excess pressure on the natural hair and scalp.

MAINTAINING YOUR EXTENSION BRAID SCULPTURE

STYLE	FIBER	SIZE OF BRAIDS	DURATION OF STYLE	FREQUENCY OF SHAMPOOING
Individual Braids	Synthetic Hair Acrylic Yarn Human Hair	Small	3 Months 3 Months 3 Months	Once a week Once a week Every 2 weeks
	Synthetic Hair Acrylic Yarn Human Hair	Medium	2 Months 2 Months 1½ Months	Once a week Once a week Once every 2 weeks
	Synthetic Hair Acrylic Yarn	Large	1 Month 1 Month 1 Month	Once every 2 weeks Once a week Once every 2 weeks
Cornrows	Synthetic Hair	Very Large	2–3 Weeks	Cleanse scalp with antiseptic and a cotton swab every day until you remove braids
Goddess Braids	Acrylic Yarn			
One-Layer Cornrows (Close to the scalp)	*Synthetic Hair Acrylic Yarn	Large	1 Month	Once every 2 weeks
Cornrows and Individual Braid Styles		Medium Small	1½ Months 2–3 Months	Once every 2 weeks Once every 2 weeks

* Human Hair is not a suitable extension fiber for cornrows.

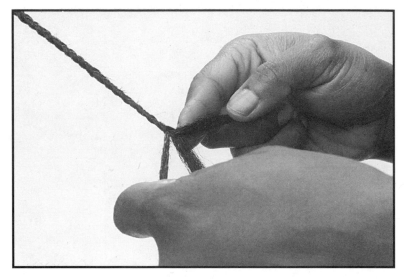

After securing the extension hair to the hair at the scalp, braid the hairpiece to the desired length.

FINISHING TECHNIQUES

It's one thing to design and create the style. It's quite another to have a finished, professional look. You want whatever natural hairstyle you have chosen to create to have a polished look. These techniques are similar to the ones that salon professionals use. I cannot stress enough that you must exercise caution and patience when trimming the braids or burning the ends. When these techniques are executed with care and concentration, you can expect the very best.

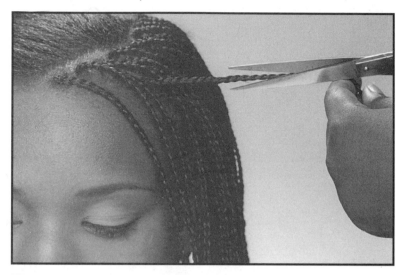

Trimming the braids is essential for a professional look. Hold the braid extended out and away from the head with one hand, take the scissors in the other hand, and, starting from the base of the braid, work your way down to the end, trimming away the stray hairs that are outside of the braid stitch.

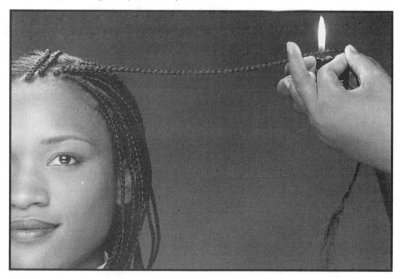

Singeing synthetic braid ends is a process that must be done with extreme care. A cape or towel should be worn over the shoulders. Hold the braid out away from the body and, using a lighter, ever so slightly touch the end of the braid.

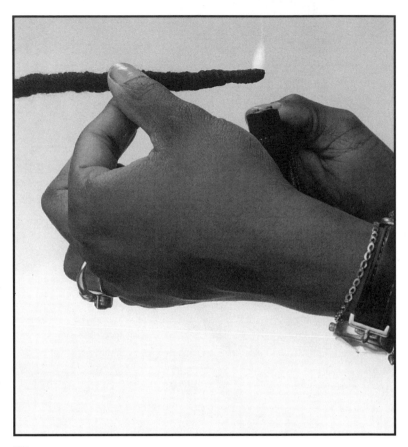

Take a lighter and burn the ends to secure the knot. The braid will melt. Blow out the flame and quickly roll the end with your index finger and thumb to make the end a smooth, slightly rounded cylinder shape. You may also roll the ends by using curling rods to achieve the same effect. *(Caution: The melted end will be very hot. Protective gloves should be worn to prevent injury to your fingers. This technique can only be used with synthetic hair and acrylic yarn.)*

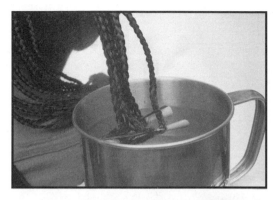

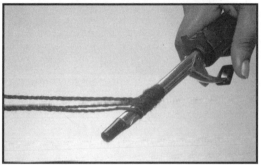

Kanekalon synthetic hair is very popular due to its light weight, soft texture, and its ability to hold a curl. Wet the ends of the braids with warm water. Use an electric curling iron set on medium and curl the wet hair ends. The hair will let off a small amount of steam while being curled.

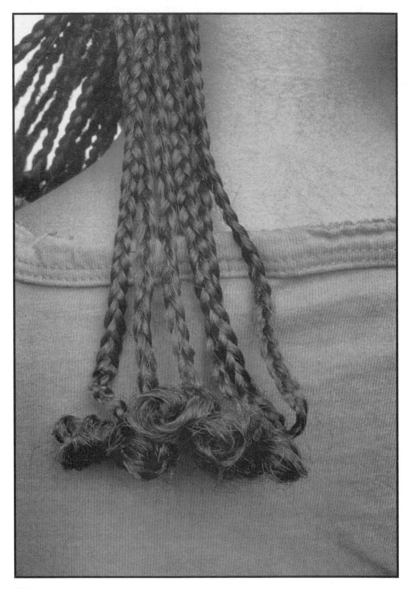

The result is beautiful curls, an elegant style, and a world-class finish.

GROOMING TECHNIQUES

One of the best things about having braided hair is that after it's washed, most times all you have to do is wait for it to dry. You don't have to think about rolling, setting, combing, brushing, or styling. Everything is done. However, whether your hair is braided naturally or with an extension fiber, all braided styles require care throughout the duration of the hairstyle.

COMING CLEAN ON STOCKING CAPS

Over the years this particular method of grooming has been passed around by word of mouth, and every time I've heard it as *gospel,* I've had to point out the lack of logic of this grooming technique. It is not a clean or healthy way to groom your braided hairstyle. *Please do not wash your hair while wearing a stocking cap!*

Let's really look at this. Here's an experiment for you to perform. Put an old stocking over a brush. Pull the stocking taut over the bristles of the brush, so they pierce the nylon a little (so the stocking will stay in place). Now brush your hair with it. When you are finished, pull the stocking cap off the brush. Any debris, oil, or dust particles that may have been in your hair are now on the stocking. If you put the stocking cap on your head, shampoo and lather up, then rinse, where is the dirt going to go? It's not going anywhere! It will be lying right on top of your braids, in the stocking cap that is pulled taut on your head. The stocking cap is supposed to keep your braids in place while you're washing your hair. If your braids are done well they will survive a weekly shampoo without a stocking cap.

SHAMPOOING YOUR BRAIDS

CORNROWS

I strongly recommend synthetic hair for cornrow hairstyles. This fiber will hold the natural hair in place, because it does not expand with the use of moisturizing shampoos and conditioners.

The style should be washed every week. Cornrows are more delicate than individual braids. Apply the shampoo directly to the braids (if the style is old or coming apart for whatever reason, dilute both the shampoo and conditioner). Massage gently in the directional flow of the braids, working up a lather. Rub your fingertips in between the rows (touching the scalp) very gently. Then rinse with water. Repeat the process twice, or as many times as you feel necessary (taking into consideration the overall age and condition of the style).

After the final rinse, apply a conditioner to the hair. You may use a leave-in conditioner, hot oil treatment, or a deep conditioner.

You may use a heating cap to deepen the conditioning action. The ultimate deep-conditioning process is the steam machine (this is an expensive machine for professional use only); it has a hood (like a dryer hood) that provides steam to the head. It opens the pores in the scalp to release any toxins, and the moist heat helps the conditioner penetrate the cuticle. I've used a steam machine for more than ten years. I would never be without one. You can simulate the effect yourself in the steam room at a gym. I don't recommend using towels. It is easy to get burned with the hot water that condenses under them. After shampooing and conditioning, gently towel-dry your hair.

Now it's time to moisturize. Apply your moisturizing hair oil to the scalp between the cornrows, and on top of the cornrows. Apply a small amount of aloe vera gel (try to mix the gel with a bit of almond oil in the palm of your hand before applying), stroking in the direction of the cornrows until it's blended into the braids.

Do not use a lot of oil or gel! If you use an excessive amount, it will cake on the braids and look horrible when it dries.

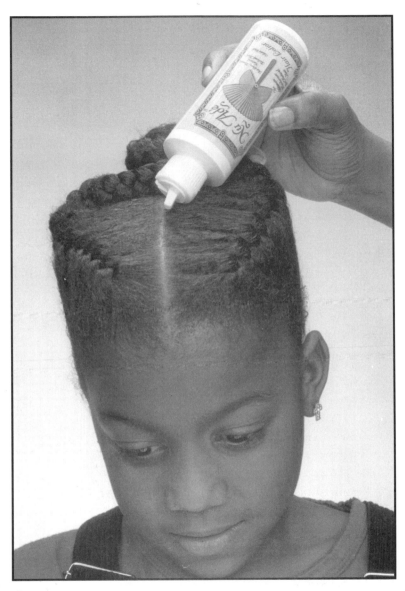

Apply moisturizing hair oil sparingly in between the cornrows.

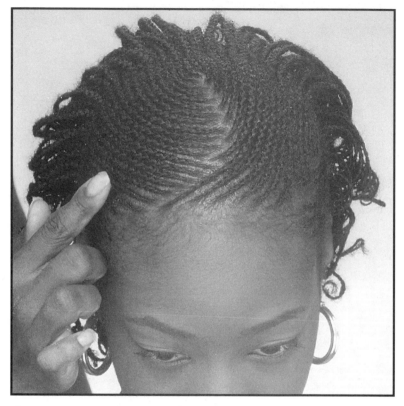

Apply a very small amount of the gel mixture to the cornrows, gently rubbing in the direction of the braids.

Tie a cotton scarf around your hair, and let it air-dry—or sit under a hood dryer. Try to schedule your home grooming during leisure time. You will then have another opportunity to really pamper yourself—and your hairstyle.

INDIVIDUAL BRAIDS

Individual braids should be washed with the same level of care.

Synthetic braids are far more durable than human-hair braids. Synthetic braids can be washed every week. (For those who work out and need to wash their hair daily, if the braids are done well this

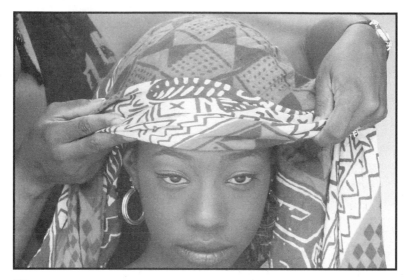

This square cotton scarf (silk can also be used) is folded into a triangle and placed around the crown of the head.

is okay. However, they will not look as nice three months later with daily shampooing, when compared to someone who shampooed once a week.) After the shampooing and conditioning process is complete, apply a moisturizing hair oil to your scalp and braids. You can air-dry your braids or go under a hood dryer.

As long as your hairstyle lasts, a light moisturizing hair oil should be used daily or as often as your natural hair texture needs it. The reason you need to do this is to take care of the new growth coming in. You want your hair to be moisturized, strong, and healthy. If you are not able to cleanse your hair and scalp (due to illness, time constraints, etc.), you can take a cotton swab and go through your scalp with an antiseptic to remove the sebum lying on the scalp. Use a product that is refreshing, with a light scent. Sea Breeze is a good choice.

Before you go to bed, tie your hair up with a cotton scarf to keep the braids from fraying while you sleep. If you tend to toss and turn, two scarves may better serve your purpose. Tie one scarf to the back, then place the second one on top and tie it to the front.

TAKING OUT YOUR BRAIDS

When you're ready to take out the braids, decide if you have the patience and the time to do it yourself—don't make it a stressful process. If you don't want to do it, have a professional do the work. Most professional natural-hair-care salons offer this service at either a flat rate or an hourly fee. If anyone involved in this process is giving you stress, leave them alone and know that the Creator provides. You'll find just the person you need. Your head will make the connection.

If you do decide to embark upon this process yourself, you will need the following tools:

- Wide-toothed comb
- Medium, small-toothed rattail comb (in the case of micro-braids, a fine hat pin–like instrument or a single wooden pick)

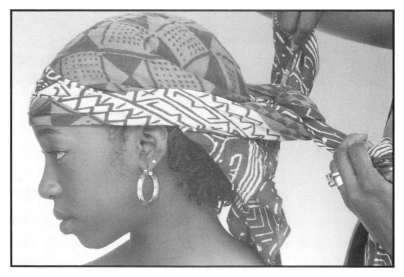

Take the two ends on either side of the head and tie them together at the back snugly. (These ends can be brought back around to the forehead and tied again to attain greater security.)

- Hair clamp, or duck-tail clips (to hold sections of your hair)
- Spray bottle containing diluted conditioner or moisturizing hair oil
- Towel for your shoulders
- Trash receptacle (for the extension braids)
- Mirror
- Music or a good video (maybe a few)

INDIVIDUAL BRAIDS

Divide the braids into small sections. Dampen each section with the diluted conditioner and hair oil (this solution softens the braids, making them easier to remove). Take three or four braids in the section, and hold them together at the ends using the medium-toothed comb (for small and medium-sized braids). Start combing out the braids, going up the length of the braid.

When you come to the portion of the braid covering the natural hair, comb through one braid at a time. Depending upon how tangled the hair is, you may have to pick each stitch apart down to the base of the braid. When the entire head is free of extensions, each base to which the braids were attached must be gently combed through before shampooing and conditioning.

CORNROWS

Taking down cornrows is a little different, because these braids lie on the scalp.

You begin by applying the diluted conditioner and/or oil to the braids, grouping a few of the ends of the braids together and using the medium-length, small-toothed rattail comb.

Gently comb up the braid until you reach the scalp. At that point each cornrow stitch must be picked apart gently with the front tooth of the comb in a downward motion.

NATURAL BRAIDS

These braids are taken down the same way. The only small difference is that the conditioning solution should work that much better, because it was developed to work on human hair.

Braids are one example of how our ancestral memory has enabled us to adorn ourselves, as well as heal the maladies brought on by our experience of slavery. These hairstyles, when properly cared for with a small investment of time, will return not only in good hair growth but also good spiritual health.

DRAMATIC PROFILE

Let me take the liberty of giving you a client profile.

Olana is experiencing a double celebration; her thirtieth birthday, and a promotion to the head of her department at work. The stress she experienced getting to the top really took a toll on her relaxed, colored hair. Olana now has bald spots where she used to have hair, and she had the choice of cutting her hair very short or hiding it under a wig. Well, Olana did not like the low 'fro look, and she never considered wearing a wig. Olana has considered braids in the past because she knows another sister across the hall who wears them, and she always looks classy. Olana's taste and style are impeccable and she dresses Afrocentrically anyway, so her choice of styles is endless. The first consideration is her alopecia (balding). Let's review Chapter One.

The chemicals (relaxer and color) severely damaged her follicles. They penetrated the cuticle, fried off the outer scales, causing a dry, flaking condition, and went into the cortex and damaged the strength and elasticity of her hair. They probably fried the sebaceous glands, too. We won't blame all of this on the chemicals, because the stress at her job was incredible. Olana's nervous system was all out of order, and the clean, smooth areas on the top of her head and around the nape of her neck were a clear indication of this. These are common areas that indicate stress-induced alopecia areata. The relaxer and color did a lot of damage, but her frayed nerves did even more.

My prescription*:

Cardiovascular exercise and yoga would be an excellent place to start. Why? An increased flow of blood and oxygen through her body would begin to nourish the papilla (hair root), and begin the healing process for the damaged nerve tissue in that area. The yoga would also help to stretch Olana's muscles after a good workout, as well as provide good meditation techniques to calm and focus her mind and spirit.

A session with a good nutritionist would pinpoint what vitamins and foods she needs to be eating to nourish her body back to health.

LET'S BREAK IT DOWN

Olana's hair regimen should start with a good moisturizing shampoo with a pH factor of 6.5, and a deep-penetrating conditioner with a steam treatment before braiding begins. Synthetic or acrylic extension hair should be used, because it would be less stressful on her natural hair.

The style should be an individual pixie or bob. These two styles are very short. The length would not go below the chin for the bob, and the pixie would be layered. The longest point would be at the earlobe, so there would be no temptation to pull the braids back or up, which would put further stress on her hairline. The fibers are very durable, so they would be able to hold up to weekly shampooing and deep conditioning. It may be more often than weekly, if she is involved in rigorous cardiovascular activities. This style would last up to three months with a "touch-up" (rebraiding) around her edges. Olana's edges are weak, and we would not want the weight of a long extension to break off any new growth in that area.

---

* I am in no way claiming to be a medical doctor, but I do know my heads.

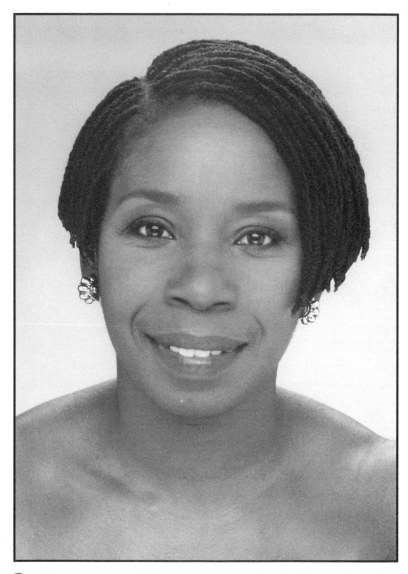

Iyanla is wearing a small Nu loc extension, bob style. This braided style is created with acrylic yarn. It is very light and durable. As it ages, it gives the wearer the appearance of having natural locs. *(Stylist, Nicole James)*

CHAPTER

FIVE

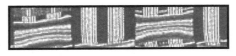

BEYOND BRAIDS

I'M ALWAYS AMAZED by the new styles that are created within the realm of natural hair. If you are tired of wearing braids, and you are clear you will not return to the "relaxed" side of things, then you are ready to go beyond braids.

Sit and look in the mirror and consider the possibilities. Think about what's comfortable and what will work for your lifestyle. Consider your jewelry and wardrobe. This may be the very incentive you need to go and add some new pieces to your collection. One thing is for sure—there are many beautiful styles to consider. They will wait patiently as you select and wear one after the other.

SHORT AND SIMPLE

Many women feel that cutting their hair down to a little more than "that much hair" serves them very well. Run your hand across your head, and it's practically "combed" for the day. Your hair still has to be groomed according to shape and texture, however, even though there's less of it.

TWO-STRANDED TWISTS

This style is a nice variation on a braided hairstyle. Depending on the length of your hair, you may create other styles as you would with individual braids. Or you may opt to leave them twisted for a period of time, then take them apart for a springy Afro look. You can also use Bantu knots. You can always get at least three styles out of having these two-stranded, single twists.

Implements needed:

- Spray bottle filled with water
- Moisturizing hair oil
- Aloe vera gel (optional)

These instructions are for a style of two-stranded twists without cornrows.

After a shampoo and conditioning, towel dry the hair until damp. Keep the spray bottle handy because you will have to re-dampen the hair as it dries.

- Oil the hair very lightly.
- Part the hair into ¼ to ½ inch sections beginning at the nape of the neck. Dampen the hair section with a very small amount of the aloe vera gel.
- Split the section in half so you have a section of hair in each hand between your index finger and your thumb. Cross one section over the other. You will be passing and trading one section of hair from your index finger and thumb to the other hand's index finger and thumb.
- Continue this crossing-over motion until you have reached the end of the twist. Divide the pieces into three sections and braid them to the end to secure the twist from unraveling.

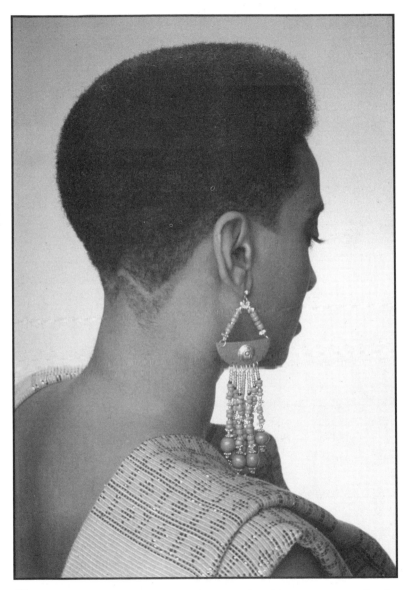

Carefree closely cropped cuts have become the ultimate statement for the time-conscious woman of the nineties. A gentle fade on the hairline, blending into a couple of inches at the top, softens the angles of the cut. A short, cropped style has to be groomed according to its texture. *(Stylist, Nilaja Yarborough)*

• When you have completed the process you should have a head full of beautiful twists. If it is your desire to have the twists lay flat on your head, tie them down with a cotton scarf.
• This style should last until you decide it's time to take it out. Often people begin to lock their hair by leaving the twists in until they begin to lock at the root. Then they start palm rolling. It can be washed and conditioned while it is twisted.

THREAD WRAPPING

This is a traditional style taken from any number of cultures across the African continent. The hair is parted off into geometric patterns, then each section is wrapped with thread to create an interconnected, three-dimensional hair sculpture. The style lasts about three weeks.

BANTU KNOTS

Rooted in traditional African styling, Bantu knots have become a popular hair sculpture. They can be worn with a formal occasion in mind, at the workplace, or in casual dress. This style may be performed with loose natural hair, relaxed hair, or with extensions.

• The sections for each knot can be made from one to three square inches or more.
• Twist the hair around if it's loose (for twists gather a few according to the square inch area), then place your index finger at the base of the twist and wrap the twist round your finger. After wrapping, tuck the end of the twist under the outer rim of its base.
• How much hair you are working with will determine the method you will use to secure the ends. If the knots are big, use bobby pins to hold in the ends. If they are medium-sized, tuck

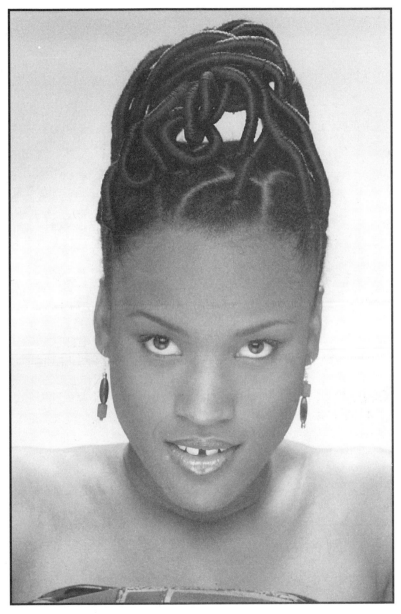

Traditional African thread wrapping. Black cotton thread was used to create this beautiful hair sculpture. *(Stylist, Amma McKen)*

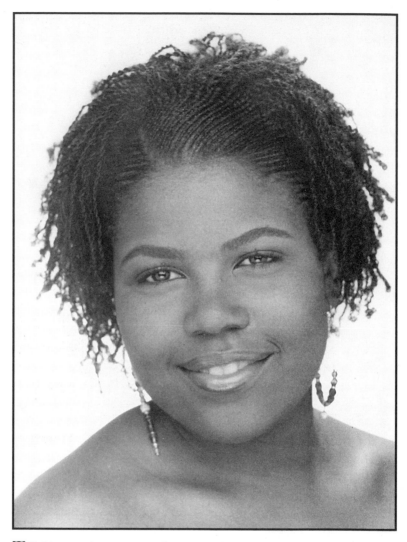

Talliah's natural cornrows and two-stranded twists can become three different hairstyles: cornrows and two-stranded twists, Bantu knots, and curly twists with cornrows.

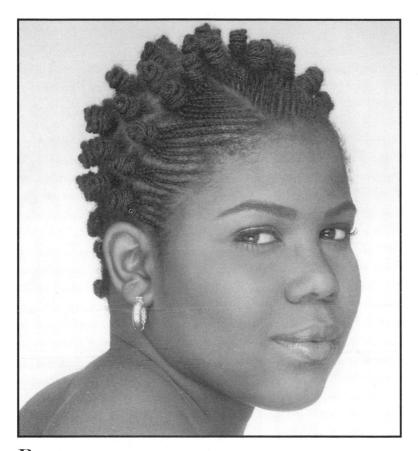

Bantu knots.

the ends in under the base, or sew them by running a needle back and forth thru the end and the base.

• Bantu knots should last about two weeks, and when they are unraveled the hair will have a springy curl. If the hair was twisted while it was damp, the curl while be very tight.

• *Note: Whenever you are working with damp hair make sure it is moisturized with a very light moisturizing oil.*

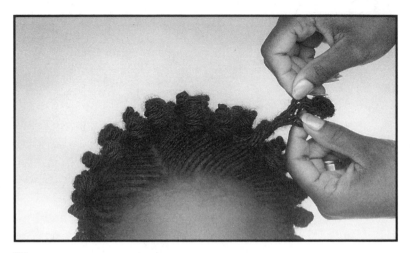

Bantu knots served to set the hair for the following style.

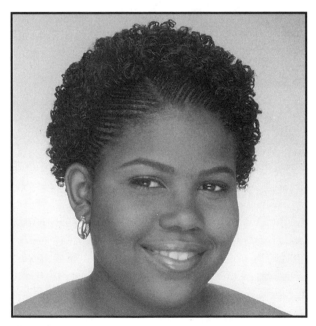

Curly twists are the end result of Bantu knots. When shampooed, the tight curls can be set to become loose curls, for yet another style. *(Stylist, Avion Julien)*

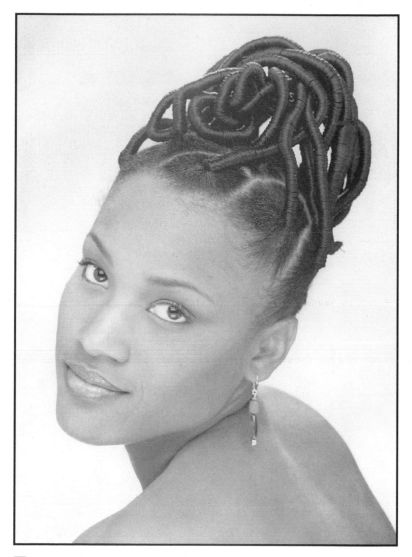

Traditional thread wrapping has always been at the foundation of adornment in Africa. Nique's hair is parted in symmetrical designs and the hair is wrapped with thread to achieve a three-dimensional sculpture, that more often than not holds a meaning of tradition for the wearer. *(Stylist, Amma McKen)*

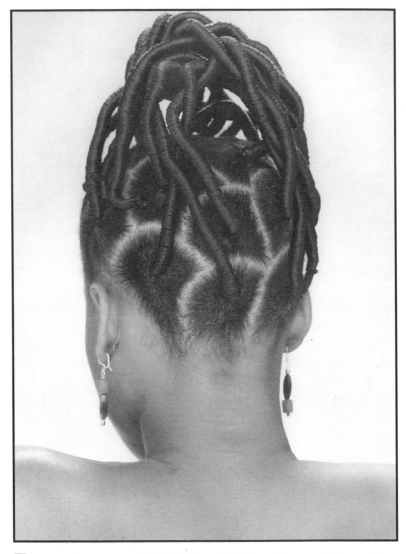

The rear view shows off the Nigerian "bridge" sculpture and the precision of Amma McKen, natural-hair-care specialist. Her artistic expertise has created wrapped hairstyles for actresses Angela Bassett and Alfre Woodard. *(Stylist, Amma McKen)*

FLAT TWISTS

Flat twists are a beautiful, quick, and easy style for almost any hair texture. They can be done with natural hair or extensions. The style lasts about two to three weeks. It is delicate, so you would need to tie it up at night. The only prerequisite is that you have a good hairline because the twist is started at the very edge of your hairline then pulled back while styling.

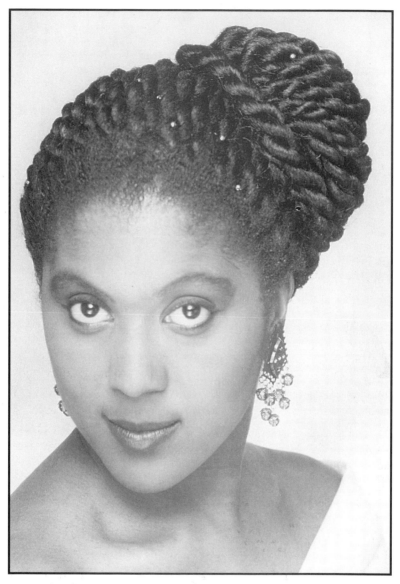

Extension flat twists are a great interim style. They last up to two weeks with very careful care. Synthetic hair is twisted into the hairline and worked backwards, picking up natural hair as it's twisted back. Each row was twisted back on the surface of Debbie's head into a spiral bun. Your hairline must be strong and healthy to wear this style. *(Stylist, Codu Thiam)*

CHAPTER

SIX

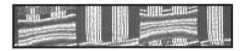

LUSCIOUS LOCS

ABOUT FOUR YEARS AGO, I was walking in Midtown Manhattan taking care of some errands for my Brooklyn natural-hair-care salon, when suddenly I noticed that it seemed like every third black person I saw had locs. Not baby locs, but locs that were mature—at least two years old. Then I took the train back home to Brooklyn, where I now noticed locs on almost every other black person. I said to myself, "Now wait, where have I been? I didn't go anywhere, where are all these mature locs coming from? Why didn't I see this before? Were all these people wearing hats or something?" I returned to the salon, and told Avion and Nicole what I had just experienced. I asked them, "Do you see what I see?" They said, "You know, Tulani, we were just saying the same thing." Locs had finally come into style.

For whatever reason, be it style, evolution, the result of a deep personal transformation to the natural, or answering an ancestral call to embrace our African aesthetic, locs are a commitment to the natural. Each one of those reasons lends support to a population of folks who are wearing locs in the nineties.

Dread locs, Nubian locs, African locs, locs, are the names used to describe the joining together of strands of curly, coiled African hair. (It has been said that the way curly, coiling African hair grows is very much like the DNA molecule, the cellular blueprint of life found in every human being.)

Certainly, locs are the real "permanent." There is no chemical restructuring of the natural hair in order to wear the style; the only requirements are patience and commitment.

Once they have grown to a certain length the process of locking is irreversible, and the length to which your hair will grow is limited only by a pair of scissors. The process is this: When hair is

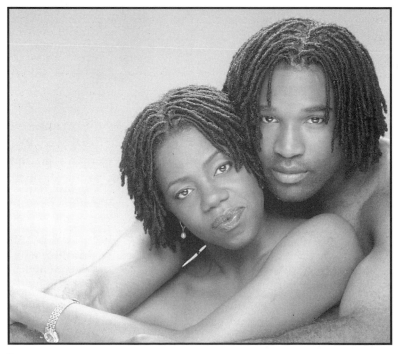

Lala and Luther have made the commitment to locs—and each other. *(Stylist, Nicole James)*

no longer combed or brushed, every strand that would otherwise come out from a normal grooming regimen, along with shedding and breakage, starts to become entwined, meshing, spiraling, coiling, and locking together, drawing into a cylinder formation that becomes "locked."

It has been four hundred years since we were brought to these shores as slaves, leaving behind on the continent of Africa a beauty aesthetic unmatched by other cultures with respect to the adornment of our heads. Again, I say the head was, and still is, a sacred place.

Starting in the cradle of civilization, ancient Khemet (now called Egypt) around 3500 B.C., locs are quite evident in drawings on Egyptian artifacts. Locs were worn by priests, and by people of prominence and royal status within the community. Locs were depicted as the hairstyles of some gods and goddesses. Isis (goddess of wisdom) and Maat (goddess of law and justice) are just two of the Egyptian deities depicted with locs.

- New York–based Master "Loctitian" Ona created her innovative Locksmyth technique after observing a drawing on an Egyptian artifact showing a loc grooming session.
- In the Old Testament, there were Israelites who followed a specific spiritual path in which they dedicated themselves to God. They were called Nazerenes. One of their practices is described in the book of Numbers, 6:5: "All the days of the vow of his separation shall no razor come upon his head . . . and shall let the locks of his hair of his head grow."
- In Nigeria, the Yoruba people declared that any child born with hair that locked automatically had spiritual prominence as a child of the Orisa (traditional religious deity and force of nature) DaDa.
- The sanctity of having one's hair locked has appeared in other cultures across the globe. Due to the variety of textures, the appearance is different from the tightly coiled loc of an African hair type. Sadhus, holy men in India, are identified by their locs. Buddhists refer to a holy man being identified by the curling of

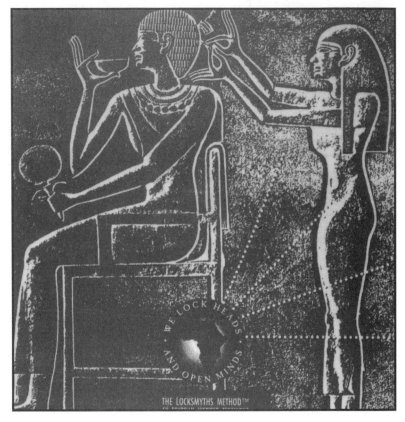

Ancient Khemetian (Egyptian) loc grooming session. *(Photo taken by Ona Osiri Maat)*

his hair. Some sculptures of the Buddha are done with the "baby loc" hairstyle.

• Rastafarians are perhaps the best known religious devotees to hair locking. They consider their hair sacred and keep it covered in public.

Those who wear locs for fashion or style reasons usually don't wear them for more than two years. Even within that context, they had to give patience and time to attain a particular length of hair. Today, just like anything else, where there is a will there is a way. These folks no longer have to wait any long length of time to attain a mature loc look. If your money is long enough, your locs can be as well. You can now buy extension locs that will flow down your back, and only you and your natural-hair-care specialist will know you did not grow them.

Most people have been drawn to locs because of their astounding beauty, once they have reached a significant length. The fluidity and beauty of an impeccably groomed head of long locs is a sight to behold. First of all, most folks are not used to seeing African hair at any length below the shoulders. Secondly, it's no secret that locs take a lot of time and effort to groom. That level of care and attention is immediately evident to anyone, viewing a well-locked head of hair.

My first set of locs grew to the middle of my shoulder blades before I cut them. My grandmother was astonished. She kept asking me if my locs were really my hair. She was used to my bead cap (microbraids and beads). Because my locks were also beaded, it never occurred to her that my locs were not braids until they started to grow past my shoulders. She knew I had never worn long extensions, so she began to wonder if I was getting carried away with the "extension look."

My locks were cut as part of the initiation ceremony into the Orisa priesthood. My grandmother just knew I was a fool. I think she thought my hair would never grow to that length again. When my daughter and I started locking our hair, all she could say, in her Montserrat accent, was, "I'm just watchin' you, ya know" and smile. Our locs have become a source of pride for her. My joy would be to start her on locs!

When making the decision to loc your hair, you first must give the issue deep thought and consideration. These are permanent. You will not be taking these out. To go to another style you will have to cut off the locked hair. Locs are truly the "real" permanent. In their initial stage of development, locs are seldom more than three to four inches long. These "buds" can take anywhere from three to six weeks or two to four months.

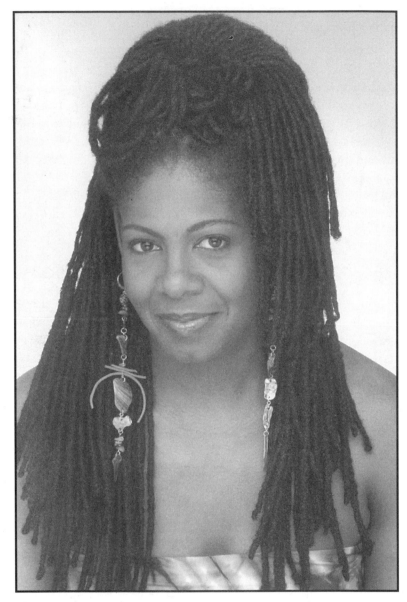

Amma McKen's locs were started six years ago. Her locs are always impeccably groomed. Grooming with moisturizing hair lotion creates a healthy sheen
and provides moisture to her locs. *(Stylist, Tulani Kinard)*

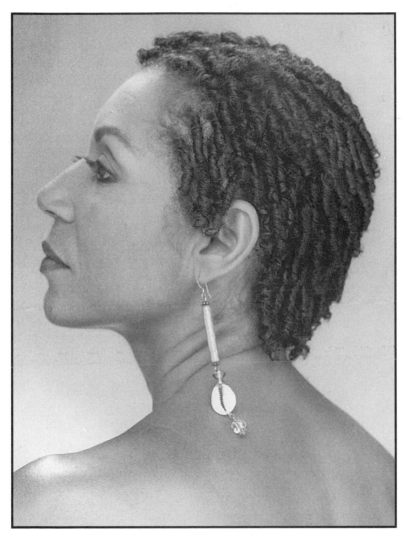

Muntu's locs are in their initial stages of growth and development. Her hair is wavy and it will not stay twisted using the same techniques that are used to loc hair growing in a tight curl pattern. A comb-twisting technique with a moisturizing hair oil and gel will set the locs. This will last until the hair gets wet. *(Stylist, Avion Julien)*

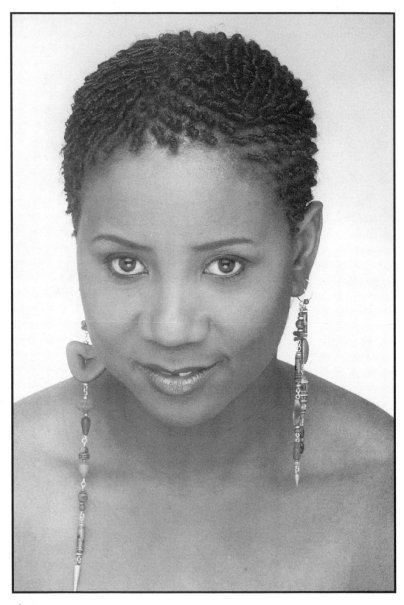

Amma has comb-coiled baby locs. Her hair is approximately an inch long. This short comb-twist will last about two weeks, or until it becomes wet. *(Stylist, Nicole James)*

After the sixth month, the wearer has become very comfortable touching and twisting his or her hair. For some it becomes a part of self-grooming, for others it is a source of pacification, or acquaintance with their hair. By the time the locs reach the length that would touch your neck, fall in your face, rub against your skin, the wearer is well acquainted, protective, proud, and in love with his or her locs.

We are moving toward the understanding that anytime an African-inspired hair sculpture is performed, an ancestral transmission has taken place. No Eurocentric hairstyle will ever attract on a daily basis the level of attention, adoration, and appreciation for living, wearable art as will an Afrocentric hairstyle. It does not matter if it's an Afro, braids, or locs.

For women in the initial stages of budding locs, issues of femininity are broached by those who believe a woman must have long hair. Negative imagery over the years has taken root in many of the elders in our families, and they will probably think you have lost your mind. The people on your job may have been just getting used to braids, or in many cases feel that anything other than a chemical straightener is totally unprofessional, and could jeopardize your ability to earn a living. Depending upon where you live in this country, it may also be an unpopular way for you to look.

I can tell you, No Lye, that I've just about seen it all. But I'm here to testify that, if you go on through, because you've determined that locs are right for your growth and development as a person of African descent, you won't be sorry. There is a sense of having come to a place of satisfaction, security, and self-confidence that exists in wearing locs. Once you have worn them to a level of maturity (three years or more), then decide to cut them off, two things will happen: (1) you will never go back to altering the natural structure of your hair again; and (2) a sense of freedom about your beauty will exist, to the point of being comfortable enough with yourself to wear any natural hairstyle with a regalness that exudes self-esteem and constantly affirms who you are.

NUBIAN LOCS

The texture of your natural hair will determine a number of things:

- How long it will take for your hair to loc
- What technique is best suited for your texture
- Whether you need extensions or a wrapping technique to help loc it

HOW LONG IT TAKES AND WHETHER OR NOT TO LOC

As a rule, the tighter the curl pattern of your hair, the easier it is to loc. It will usually take about six months on the average to get a "sho' nuff" loc.

If your hair is wavy and soft, it will take a very long time for your hair to loc. There are alternative methods, like having individual braids done all over your head and letting them stay in until they loc. Again, texture makes a difference—if your hair's really soft, it could take a year or more.

Salon techniques, like Sister Locks, will definitely create the environment for your hair to loc. It will still take time, but frustration about having your hair unravel and look unkempt will be put to rest.

Hair that is between curly and wavy will lock, but it needs to be left alone. There are ways you can aid the locking process: (1) leaving in individual braids; (2) leaving in two-stranded twists; or (3) setting the whole head in palm-rolled or comb-coiled locs, then attaching a Nu Loc braid extension to each section. This is an acrylic-yarn extension-braid technique. It is left on for approximately three months, then removed. At that time your loc should have a strong base. You can then either opt to retwist the loc and reapply the Nu Loc extension for another three

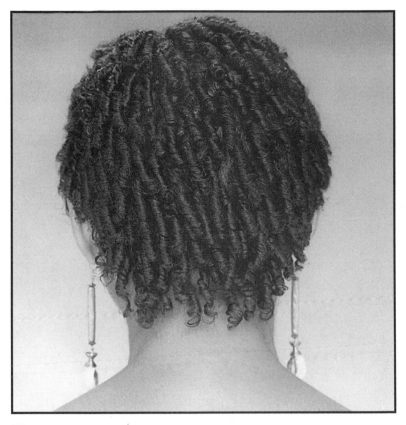

This is a rear view of Muntu's locs. The softness of her hair texture will extend the period of time it takes her hair to loc—from six months to a year. *(Stylist, Avion Julien)*

months, or start palm rolling what you have and go on from there.

Two of the benefits of applying the Nu Loc extensions are: (1) you can prepare your family and friends for what your locs will look like; and (2) you can determine the length of the Nu Locs, especially if you want to be able to have enough length to vary the style of them.

Thread wrapping is another alternative to consider. Your hair

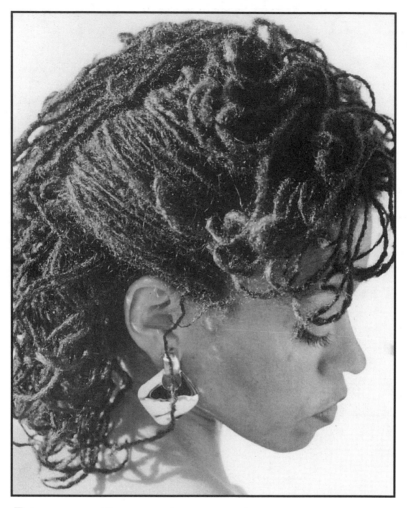

JoAnne Cornwell's Sister Locks technique enables those who have a soft texture to loc their hair much sooner than the prescribed six months to a year. These "microlocs" have tensile strength and styling versatility. *(Groomed and styled by Dr. JoAnne Cornwell)*

can be set into the loc formation, then each loc can be thread wrapped to give support to the locking process.

In each of the aforementioned extension techniques, the hair can be washed and conditioned on a regular basis.

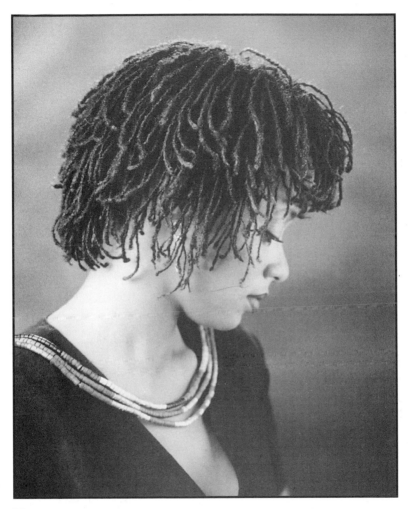

Photo of Sister Locks.

MAKING THE TECHNIQUES YOUR OWN

There are three techniques for beginning your locs yourself. Many people have met with great success using them. I recommend that even if you decide to start and groom your own locs that

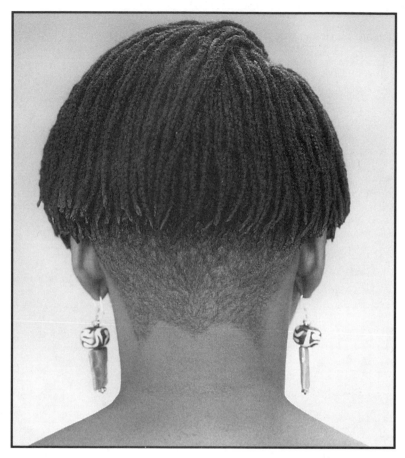

This is a rear-view shot of Iyanla'a "Nu Locs." Prior to the application of the acrylic yarn extensions, her hair was sectioned and twisted for locs. The Nu Loc extensions were then braided onto the loc twists. While waiting for the locs to grow to a certain length, she has both a variety of styles to wear and help in the "locking" process. *(Styled by Nicole James)*

you should schedule an appointment to have professional treatment at least once every couple of months. It's always relaxing and often a luxury to have your locs groomed by a professional loctitian.

These three techniques—Palm rolling, Braiding, and Two-stranded twists—are started the same way. You must part your hair in small ½ inch sections. Whatever technique you decide to use should be determined by the texture and curl pattern of your hair.

If your hair has a very tight curl pattern, you should use the palm rolling technique. If your hair has a loose, wavy pattern and is almost straight, braiding would be the best technique. If you have a curl pattern between very curly and wavy, then the two-stranded twist would work best for you.

TOOLS

Comb
Clips
Spray bottle
Gel (aloe vera or light, nonalcohol commercial gel)
Moisturizing hair oil
Cape, towel, or other covering for your clothing
Mirror

TACKLING THE TECHNIQUES

Do not under any circumstances use beeswax to start your locs. This product will hold your locs together but will be next to impossible to wash out when it's time to cleanse your hair. It will leave your locs looking very dull, in addition to attracting and holding dust and debris.

For all techniques, whether it be palm rolling, braiding, two-stranded twisting, or any other salon techniques, your hair should be prepared by shampooing it with a pH-balanced shampoo, followed with a hot oil moisturizing treatment. (See Chapter Three for proper shampooing procedures.)

Towel-dry your hair, to eliminate excess water, but leave the hair damp. Part the hair on a horizontal slant, and take equal sections from within the horizontal part to make a cylinder loc.

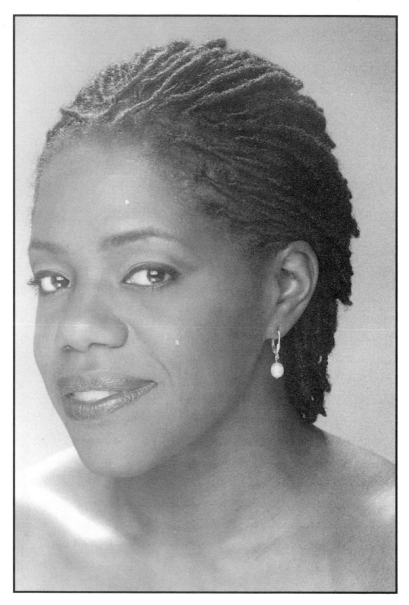

Lala's locs are groomed with Nu Crown Hair Oil. The oil is light and mois-turizing, and gives her locs a healthy sheen. Beeswax or any other heavy wax or petroleum-based product sits on the loc, causing it to look dull, especially after shampooing. *(Stylist, Nicole James)*

Always take into consideration the condition of your hair. If your hair tends to be very oily, then a hot oil treatment is not really your best choice for a conditioner. Refer to Chapter Three to determine the best types of products for your hair.

PALM ROLLING

You need at least three inches of natural hair for palm rolling. Your texture can be soft, medium, or coarse, and your curl pattern should be more inclined toward a springy, medium-to-tight curl for this technique to retain its shape and form.

Start at the base of the neck and take a small section of hair. Part off a horizontally slanted row. Make equal, small section parts on the row. They may be little box-, diamond-, or triangle-shaped parts.

Put a little gel (and I do mean a little) on each section. Place the section of hair in the crevice that is at the base of your fingers, just

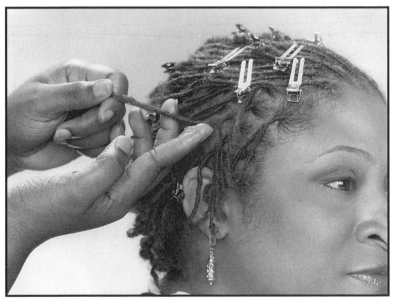

Monette's hair is sectioned and gel is applied to the hair to help the loc hold its form after it is palm-rolled.

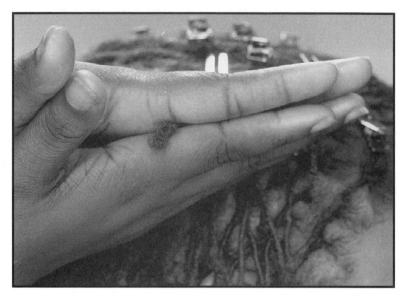

The loc is placed between the right and left palms and rolled. This technique brings all the loose and stray hairs into the loc, to solidify its cylindrical structure.

above the palm of your left hand. Take your right hand, and place the base of your palm in the middle of the crevice of the left hand (where your fingers begin), and roll the right hand down the left-hand palm until the fingertips of the right hand come down to the base of the left palm.

Twist the loc around with your fingertips in a clockwise direction (or counterclockwise; it depends on whether you are right-handed or left-handed), lay it down against the scalp, place a clip on it to hold it in place. Proceed to the next section.

Work your way up through the back of your head until you get to the front. Keep your spray bottle handy; you will need to keep your hair damp until you are finished.

BRAIDING

You can determine the size of your locs by the size you choose to make your braids. Make equal sections all over your head. Your sections can be diamonds, squares, pyramids, or circles. Apply a small amount of gel to each section. Using an underhanded stitch, braid each section to the very end. Don't leave anything unbraided. Upon completion, you can set your hair in rollers. Actually, styling it in some way will help to keep the braid intact. Six months down the road—after bi-weekly grooming, shampooing, and conditioning—the locking process should be well on the way. As the hair begins to fuzz and fray then the palm-rolling technique can be used to pull in the loose hairs and continue the locking process.

TWO-STRANDED TWIST

This technique follows the same format as braiding, except that when you part off the hair in sections, instead of making three new sections from that, you just make two. Apply a little gel, and begin crossing each strand section over the other until you've worked

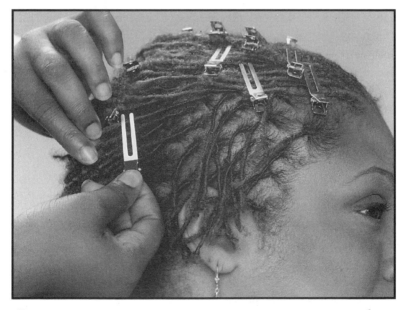

Clip the loc to hold it in place while the hair is drying. You have the choice of air-drying the locs or sitting under an electric dryer hood at a medium temperature.

your way down to the end of the twist. Toward the end of the twist, approximately two inches from it, separate the two sections into three and braid it out to finish it off.

SALON TECHNIQUES

Comb Coiling and Sister Locks are two professional techniques that can be used for two of the most difficult types of hair to lock. Very short hair and soft, wavy hair work well with comb coiling. Hair that is naturally straight or relaxed can now be started and groomed for locking using the Sister Lock technique. These two techniques give a very refined look to these textures.

COMB COILING

This beginner's loc look lasts about three weeks. The technique can be performed on hair that is as short as one inch, or as long as four to five inches.

The hair is parted, then sectioned. A small amount of gel is used, and each section of hair is coiled by placing the front teeth of a small-toothed comb at the scalp, and twisting downward to the ends of the hair. You cannot wash your hair if you want the style to last for three weeks. Be careful not to get it wet in the shower, wear a shower cap to prevent this. You can cleanse your scalp with a cotton swab doused with an antiseptic, however. Go in between each part with the wet cotton swab.

SISTER LOCKS

If you had chemically straightened hair and want to start locking your hair, we used to tell folks they had to cut off the chemically altered hair and start with the new growth. Now with the innovative technique of Sister Locks, developed by Dr. JoAnne Cornwell, the previously unattainable is now within your reach.

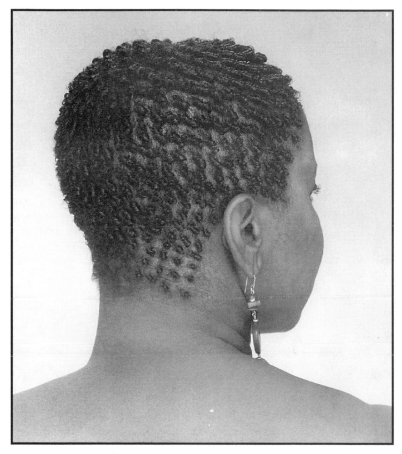

Rear view of Amma's comb-coiled baby locs. This style is ideal for those who have a close-cropped, natural cut and want a little styling variety. It's also a great way to show off a great-shaped head. *(Stylist, Nicole James)*

This technique is also excellent for naturally curly textures. This is also known as "microlocking."

The Sister Locks technique involves backward braiding—moving from the tip toward the roots of a section of hair, while looping the strands into a uniform pattern. This looping is accomplished

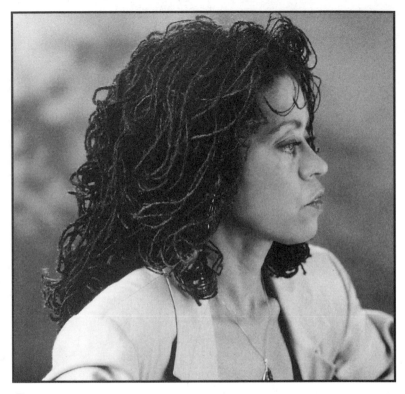

JoAnne's locs are over four years old (measure the growth with the photo earlier in the chapter). The only requirement for having locs like these is time.

by using a special tool designed to achieve a very fine loc. The microlocs can be styled in medium-to-long-length styles that involve setting the locs on rods, or using mousses, gels, and/or setting lotions for looks that previously were only attainable through the use of micro extension braids. This technique definitely requires a professional's skill; it is not something you should attempt to do yourself. This method is about four years old, and has proven very successful.

SHAMPOOING YOUR LOCS

BABY LOCS

If your hair is curly, follow this regimen for one to three months until your locs have established a base. If your hair is soft, it would take closer to three to six months.

The first time your hair is groomed into a loc style (unless it is braided), you should wait approximately three weeks before shampooing it. At that time, the loc sections will need to be retwisted.

During the three weeks before you shampoo, you can cleanse your scalp with an antiseptic. Sea Breeze is very popular. You can also use herbal rinses that are astringent, such as rosemary, sage, and rosehips (see page 133 for recipes). Dip a cotton ball or swab into the antiseptic solution. Rub it on the scalp, through the parted sections of the entire head. This should provide relief for any scalp discomfort.

When it's time to shampoo, wet the head, and apply the shampoo. Massage the scalp very gently. Try not to break up the loc sections. Rinse with warm water. Shampoo two to three times, depending on your hair's texture. If very soft, wash only once. Towel-dry gently, and apply a hot oil or herbal rinse conditioning treatment. Wait the specified time, and thoroughly rinse the conditioner out of your hair. Again, towel-dry gently or let air-dry.

MATURE LOCS

After eighteen months to two years the locs have reached the beginning stage of their maturity. At this stage there should be an inch worth of new growth every three to four months, and their total length should be four to six inches. Mature locs can be washed every day if necessary, as long as they are conditioned and oiled to combat dryness and the loss of moisture.

Every time they are shampooed you have the opportunity to retwist the locs or leave the new growth untwisted. There are those who choose not to retwist their locs after they have reached a length of ten to fourteen inches. I am one of those folks. I stopped retwisting my roots on a bi-weekly basis when my hair was twelve inches long. I brush the new growth and apply a super-moisturizing oil to the locs before styling. The loose hair is soft and cotton-like; the lock is a soft sponge of tightly woven hair. Together they appeal to my love of the way my hair was when I was a little girl and the way it is now with locs.

To wash mature locs, wet hair, apply shampoo, then gently massage into the scalp and hair. Rinse, lather, and repeat the process. Apply the appropriate conditioner, leave in for the predetermined time, and rinse. You may opt to use a leave-in conditioner or an herbal rinse. Afterwards, apply a light conditioning oil. The hair is now ready for grooming.

HAIR PREPARATIONS

Pomades—hair grease, Vaseline, or other petroleum-based hair preparations—are not good for your locked hair, since they are very difficult to wash out. They do not break down in hot water. They coat the cuticle, preventing it from opening during any cleansing regimen. The weight of these products will clog the pores in the scalp, inhibit natural flaking and cleansing, and cause the sebaceous glands to malfunction. All of these effects will lead to horrific dandruff and scalp problems. Light oils, which contain natural moisturizers, are best. They break down easily, and they don't cause buildup in the scalp or locs.

REFRESHING RINSES AND CONDITIONING OILS

Herbal and fruit rinses are wonderful because they strengthen the hair. There is a list of rinses in the recipe section in the list provided below. They are safe and easy to prepare. Choose according to your needs. These rinses are applied last, and unless specified, you can use them as your would a leave-in conditioner. Try your hand at caring for your natural hair with these rinses and oils.

Most of these herbs are sold loose and by the ounce in health-food stores. Place about two tablespoons of the dried herb into a glass or stainless steel pot of boiling water. (Do not use aluminum; it would release harmful mineral deposits into the herbal rinse.) Cover and remove from the heat. Let the mixture steep for an hour. Make sure the mixture is not hot; room temperature is good. Strain off the herbs, and use the infused water as the last rinse after a shampoo and deep conditioning treatment.

Rosemary	Stimulates circulation, solves scalp problems, good for dandruff
Rosehip	Emollient, good for damaged hair
Sage	Strengthens the hair, has astringent and antibacterial properties
Chamomile	Brightens and highlights, provides a sheen
Horsetail	Stimulates growth, helps reduce dandruff
Nettle	Retards baldness, antiseptic, good for dandruff

FRUIT RINSES

Mix one part fruit juice to three parts water. Let them sit in the hair twenty minutes and then rinse out thoroughly.

Banana rinse	Excellent emollient, highly natural lubricant and hair conditioner; beneficial to the hair and scalp because it binds with water to hold in moisture.
Coconut milk	Natural emollient with great conditioning proteins. Helps to reduce the loss of moisture and to soften and smooth the hair.
Lemon rinse	Refreshing astringent, stimulates the scalp, dissolves sebum buildup

Apple cider vinegar	Retards dandruff, provides sheen to hair

SCALP OILS FOR LOCKED HAIR

Rosemary oil	Stimulates growth, antiseptic, good for dandruff, excellent for shine on dark-colored hair
Sage oil	Astringent, stimulates growth, kills bacteria; it is said to have the ability to darken graying hair
Jojoba oil	Smooths and conditions curly hair, good for dry scalp
Sweet almond oil	Contains vitamins E and F, good for itchy scalp, mild, and easily absorbed
Avocado oil	Rich in potassium and sulfur, vitamins A, D, and E, easily absorbed
Evening primrose oil	Moisturizes and conditions the hair
Birch oil	Antidandruff, effective in treating inflamed scalps
Calendula oil	Light and astringent. Extracted from the marigold flower, it soothes scalp and eczema problems.

COLORING YOUR LOCS

Mature locs are very difficult to color. The loc is a cylinder of hair that is constructed of layers upon layers of tightly packed strands. If you are coloring your hair a darker shade than its natural color, it will take much longer than when you did not have locs. You will probably have to use two to three times more product. If you are seeking to go to a lighter color, I strongly urge you to seek a natural-hair-care professional who specializes in coloring natural hair. Changing your natural color to a lighter shade requires lifting the darker color and redepositing the shade of your choice. It is a meticulous process that must be monitored closely. It is not something that you, or you and a friend, can do because you want to save money. If coloring is done incorrectly, you could severely damage your hair, and you will probably not end up with the color you desired.

This process is definitely a chemical procedure. It is mentioned here to support your desire to use color to enhance the beauty of your natural hair. It's only fair that I give you some information about the fact that taking your locs to a different shade is not a natural process. There are many routes you can take to dye your hair, ranging from the simplicity of henna to more complex dyes. Investigate carefully before making a decision. Vegetable dyes are all natural and the safest product. Permanent dyes give good color and can be successful in achieving the desired effect. When done correctly, the shades of color that can be achieved raise the beauty of your locs to immeasurable heights.

This is a historical observation. Just sit back and think, or remember, how things have been. I have observed a cycle of five transitions that have taken us to our current level of adornment and healing of our heads, from the straightening comb and chemical straighteners to the Afro and other natural cuts, and on to braids (natural and extension styles) and next to the beauty of locs.

Who would have guessed that, as we approach the next millennium, locs would have almost equal footing with the established, traditional forms of black hair care? Locs truly are a process of patience, self-examination, and awareness of the African-American community. However, with careful instruction, encouragement, and—let's not forget—the right products, you will have luscious locs before long.

I'm just watchin' you, ya know?

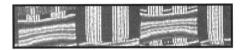

ADORNING THE
NATURAL HEAD

PEOPLE WITH DARK-COLORED HAIR, meaning brunette to black, comprise more than 70 percent of the world's population—including African, Asian, and Latino peoples. People of African descent are known for the unique way we choose to adorn ourselves and our hair. Whether you're in Lagos, Nigeria, or Brooklyn, New York, there are no limits to the ways your hair can be adorned.

The natural-hair-care movement has unleashed a particular kind of freedom with respect to hair color. Color is an easy way to give yourself another look that's totally different, without doing damage to your now healthy hair.

THE NATURAL ORIGIN OF COLOR

More than 3,000 years ago, Egyptians used henna, wild berry juice, and other vegetable-derived powders to dye everything from their hair to their clothing. African groups like the Massai warriors of Kenya and their neighbors the Samburu warriors used red ochre and animal fat to create dyes for ornamentation of their bodies and hair. The Fulani, Berber, Turkana, and Dinka groups used vegetable powders for the very same purposes. In fact, every traditional African tribe made some form of dye from indigenous plants.

The coloring process doesn't take a lot of time, and unless they want to lift (go to a lighter shade) the color of their hair, most folks opt to do the process themselves. People have become fearless in their experimentation with what they believe will enhance their beauty and make them feel good. I have *never* seen so many blond heads in my life, and because of the variety of color tones in our complexions, we can go a lot of places with color from just a hint or a highlight to a full head of color.

The best results are attained when the color choice is complementary to one's complexion, and the type of style in which the hair will be worn. A general rule that you can follow is: The lighter your hair color, the darker your skin will appear; the darker your hair color, the lighter your skin will appear. For really bold and outrageous colors, consider all of the above—and be armed with attitude.

Before you decide to change your natural hair color to a shade that is dramatically different, take a trip to a wig salon. There you will be able to try on as many different colored wigs as you like, and feel comfortable with a hair color that is going to be complimentary to your complexion and enhance your beauty.

Generally, if your hair is in good condition and you are staying within your color family, there are a few methods of coloring your hair that you can feel comfortable with doing to your own hair. Please do not hesitate to seek the expert advice of a professional colorist if:

- your hair is weak
- you are lightening your color, i.e., going from dark brown to blond, or black to ash brown
- you have mature locs and you want an even color from your roots to the tip of your locs, especially when lightening the color.

If you decide to use professional services, here are some tips to use in evaluating their level of expertise.

- You should have a consultation about what you would like to achieve.
- They should inquire about your hair history.
- A careful scalp examination should be made. If you have scratches or any type of sore or abrasion, the color service should not be done.
- They should give you a patch test on your arm the day before the actual service to determine if you are allergic to the product that will be used.
- They should provide a cape to protect your clothing and ask you to remove all jewelry.
- Remove any dye stains that may have occurred on your neck, hairline, and ears.

Following are some basic facts you need to understand before jumping off into the kingdom of color. If you remember what we learned in Chapter One about the biochemical makeup of a hair strand, you'll zoom through this section with flying colors!

YOUR PROCESS—GENERAL TIPS FOR COLORING YOUR HAIR

Patience is the key word in this situation. If you can deep condition your hair a few times prior to the actual coloring process, it will only enhance the look of the finished color. Your hair can never have enough moisture, especially when it is being colored. Implements needed:

- 2 towels
- 1 cape
- Product
- Minute timer
- Shampoo and conditioner
- Plastic gloves
- Mirror
- Stain remover (any well-stocked beauty supply store should have it)
- Table for your implements near a sink. Put some newspaper on the floor for spills.

1. Examine your scalp in the mirror to make sure there are no scratches, sores, or abrasions. You could develop serious complications if the coloring product infects any small or large open wound on your head.

2. Give yourself a patch or skin test. The label's instructions direct you on how to do so. Follow them to the letter.

3. Make 4 large sections of hair. On the crown, where the sections meet, make a circular section approximately 5 inches in diameter.

4. Apply the color to this area first. This section of the head has the least porous hair and takes the longest time to absorb color. Carefully work your way out and around the head. In each section, work your way from the inside to the out. The hairline should be the last area done because it is the most porous and absorbs color very quickly.

5. Be aware of the time it takes to complete the application of the color. Do not go over the specified time.

6. Rinse the hair with warm water until the water runs clear.

7. Shampoo the hair 2 times, then apply conditioner.

8. Towel dry or blow dry on a low heat setting.

HENNA DYES

Coloring your hair with a henna dye is the most natural—and the least damaging—way to alter your natural color. There are two types of henna. One is a pure vegetable dye, and the other is a chemical mixture of pure henna and metallic salts. Natural henna comes in powder form and is activated by hot water, to form a paste that is then applied to the hair. The henna/metallic salt product can be either a powder or a liquid. Traditionally, it has been used not only as a dye, but also as a conditioner because it helps swell the cuticle, giving the hair a thicker appearance. Generally, it should not be used without a deep conditioner, because it can dry out the scalp and hair shaft.

Try adding a little olive oil and an egg to the paste. This not only enhances the conditioning properties but the oil makes the paste smoother and will replenish any oils depleted in the coloring process.

If you repeat the coloring process two to three times, the henna creates a coating on the outer layer of the hair shaft. This coating does two things: 1) it releases you from having to color every three-four weeks since it lasts about six to eight weeks; 2) It adds body to the hair with every application. You should use a deep conditioning treatment if you are shampooing once a week. It will bring up the luster and shine of the henna coatings. (Note: You should do a strand test on gray hair to see if it will take the color.)

HOW TO USE ORGANIC HENNA

Many companies manufacture henna, in a variety of colors, including a clear henna if you just want the conditioning effects and to add body to the hair.

1. Check the scalp for scratches and sores.
2. Use gloves for the mixing and application process.
3. Follow directions on the bottle to the letter.

4. As we stated earlier, you can add an egg and some olive oil to the mixture to enhance the conditioning properties and smoothness of the product.

5. If you have decided that using henna will be your method of coloring and conditioning, invest in an inexpensive blender to make the mixing process that much smoother.

TEMPORARY COLOR

Temporary hair colors are the least harmful of all the commercial dyes. These products coat the outer layer of the hair shaft with color. The color disappears after one shampoo and conditioning.

SEMIPERMANENT COLOR

Semipermanent dyes are chemically based products, and tend not to leave hair as dry as permanent dyes. Their molecules are strong and small enough to penetrate the outer layer (the cuticle) of the hair shaft to deposit color, but they do not go into the cortex (the next layer that actually determines the color of the hair). Because these dyes do not penetrate the cortex of the hair shaft, the color will gradually fade with each shampoo. Semipermanent color can last four to six weeks.

DEMIPERMANENT COLOR

Demipermanent colors are designed to last longer than the semipermanent products. They are fairly new in the color business. Demipermanents are also marketed as "long-lasting colors," "semipermanent—no ammonia," "no peroxide," and "no-lift" (nonbleaching). However, the product is slightly stronger than the "semipermanent" products. The rule is do a patch and strand test, then proceed with caution. If you're looking for longevity with color, and you don't want the absolute permanence of stronger dyes, then give these a try.

PERMANENT DYES

Permanent dyes are made up of colored dye compounds mixed with a soapless detergent. When you purchase a brand name permanent color product, there are usually two bottles in the product. One bottle is a dark liquid, and the other a clear or creamy liquid made of hydrogen peroxide. When the color compound is mixed with the hydrogen peroxide it reacts with the oxygen in the hydrogen peroxide solution. This reaction forms large molecules of the new color that you would like the color of your hair to be. These molecules penetrate the outer layer (cuticle) and deposit themselves into the second layer (the cortex). When the process is completed the natural pigment has been replaced with the new color.

The porosity level of your hair will determine how quickly the color will be absorbed. Low porosity hair will take much longer because the large molecules of color will have to penetrate more layers of cuticles, or more tightly packed cuticles. High porosity hair will absorb the color very fast, and the chance for uneven coloring is much greater because of the high speed of absorption.

If you are thinking of changing your hair color to a lighter shade, I strongly recommend that you seek a professional hairstylist (a "colorist") who specializes in color.

In the process of going from a darker to a lighter shade, your natural color must be lifted (removed) and the new color deposited into the hair shaft. *The process is extremely stressful to the hair, and therefore I do not recommend it, if you are seeking a natural approach to caring for your hair.* Naturally dark brown or black hair, when lightened to blond, will pass through nine levels of color: black, dark brown, light brown, red, red-gold, orange, yellow-orange, yellow, and pale yellow. This process can be stopped at any point, but again you need the expertise of a colorist to determine where you should end the lifting process.

Coloring becomes fairly easy when changing your natural color to a darker shade. However, in all cases, the scalp and hair shaft become dry after the coloring process. A deep conditioning treatment will be needed every time the hair is shampooed, and a light oil with a high moisturizing content is recommended for daily maintenance.

A WORD OF CAUTION

If you have a chemical straightener in your hair and have been using henna, but now are thinking of changing to a commercial, chemical permanent dye, you must be very careful. If you choose an aniline dye (most of your major product manufacturers such as Revlon and Clairol use anilines), you must first remove the henna/metallic salt from the hair shaft. This is not an easy procedure, but it *must* be done. The chemical reaction between metallic salt present in the henna and the aniline dye will react one of several ways. It could cause the hair not to accept new color, destroy your natural hair color, quickly emit a horrible odor, melt the hair shaft, or any combination of the above.

Get a colorist to remove the henna/metallic salt from the hair shaft. This procedure is extremely drying, and very stressful to the hair. This type of henna can also make chemical straightening next to impossible to achieve. So, before starting any new hair-care regimen, style, or product, think about the potential results. And, always read labels with *great care*.

ADORNING YOUR NATURAL HEAD

BEADS

My first experience adorning a braided hairstyle was working with beads. To witness the beauty and majesty of a head full of semi-precious stones in motion always gives me chills. I realize, though, that most people are really not into wearing a full head of beads. They may only want a few to accent their braids or locs.

The smaller the beads, the less they weigh. If they are glass or semiprecious stones they lend a certain air of elegance. The size of the hole in the bead is 6.0 millimeters, so if you are adorning braids or locs, they have to be very small to fit through. If the braids or locs you wear are not that small, you can sew the beads on, and never have to worry about them falling off. They will remain secure through many grooming sessions.

Don't worry about beads matching your outfits. The more creative the bead adornment, the more people seem to appreciate the creative expression, rather than the apparel "match."

HOW TO APPLY BEADS TO YOUR BRAIDS (OR LOCS)

These instructions are for small braids or locs, but can be easily adapted for larger ones. You will need the following materials to bead your braids:

Beads
(Decide how many braids you are actually going to bead, and how many beads you are going to put on each braid.)
Button and Carpet Thread/Hair-Weaving Thread
(The B&C thread and needles can be purchased at any sewing notions store.)
Beading Wire
Scissors

PROCESS

• Cut a piece of thread 12 inches long and double it (if you want to accommodate more beads, then make it longer). Don't

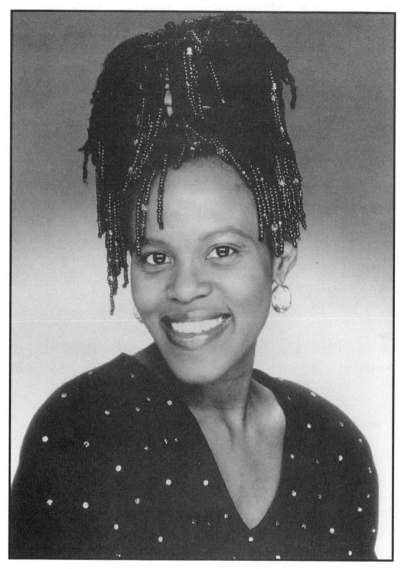

Tulani's beaded locs.

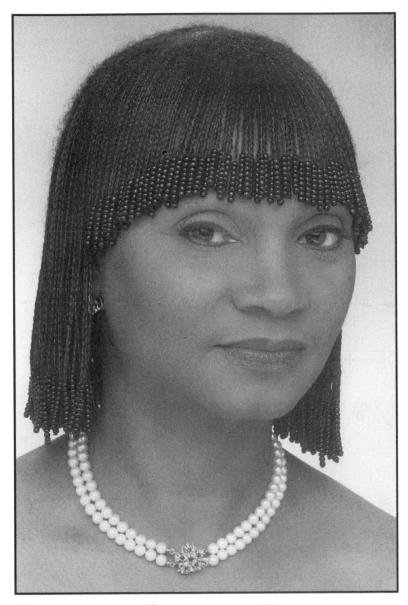

This classic interpretation of the Khemetic style of Cleopatra is known as a "bead cap" today. Black glass beads adorn the microbraids. The gentle pull of the beads collectively acts as a stimulator for hair growth. This style can last up to four months. Regular shampooing and conditioning will not disturb the beads. *(Stylist, Avion Julien)*

make it much longer, though. The length of the string and the weight of the beads would make it more difficult to manage easily.

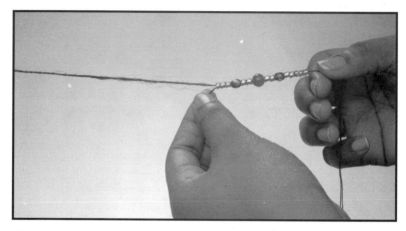

Take the end of the braid and place it through the open loop of the beaded thread.

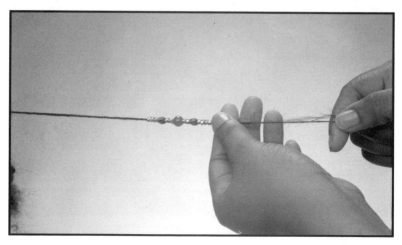

Slide beads up on to the braid.

• Place a bead on the ends of the thread and secure a knot around the bead.

• Cut a piece of beading wire 4½ inches long, and bend it in half. Thread the wire through the loop part of the doubled thread, and fold the wire together so you now have a double needle point. Twist the point so that the two ends won't come apart. You now have a needle.

• Take the needle and put it through the holes of the beads, sliding them down the thread. When you have beaded enough, untwist the wire needle and take the loop, open it, and put the end of the braid through the loop.

• Slide the beads up the thread to the very end of the braid, and push the beads up onto the braid. Loop the end of the braid up around the bead, and wrap a piece of thread about four inches long around the braid four times. Make a slip knot, tie a knot over it, and cut the end of the thread so it is not visible. Slide the remaining beads down the thread.

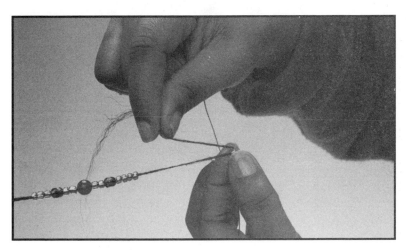

Loop the end of the braid up around the bead and wrap, slip-knot, and tie it off. *(Stylist, Tulani Kinard)*

SCULPTING BRAIDS AND LOCS

BRAIDS

There are many wonderful things that can be done with the ends of your braids and locs. Whether you're working with natural hair or synthetic or acrylic fibers, it is always possible to style the ends in a variety of fabulous ways.

Braids are often "texturized," meaning that their ends are placed on hair rods, the rods dipped into hot water, and then towel-dried.

There is an elegance created when one layer of cornrowed styles resolves into a crown. Or when a blend of natural hair and yarn (acrylic fiber) is used to create alluring hair sculpture. The ends of cornrows can be braided together into larger braids, and then entwined together and wrapped around into a bun. To change the look, single braids can be taken out, and a crimp can be put in with a curling iron and then styled into a french roll. The roll will have more depth because of the curl.

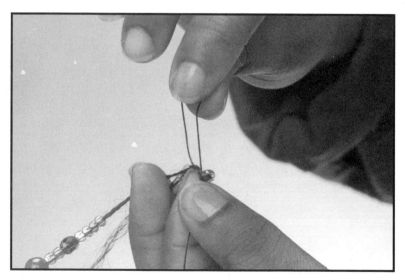

Take the hanging end of the yarn (end of the loop) and pull it back through the loop.

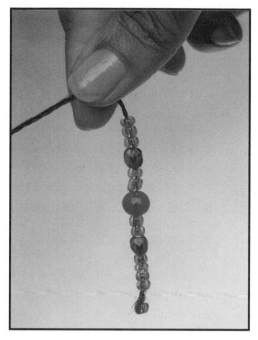

Pull the yarn through the loop and tighten Tie a small knot on top of the slip knot and cut the yarn end.

LOCS

Adorn your locs! Texturizing is one of the easiest ways to enhance the beauty of your locs. Beads, thread wrapping, rolling, and sculpting can also be done to locked hair.

Texturizing Techniques

The only criteria for using any of these techniques is having mature locs. If you have 18 months worth of growth, you're good to go!

Bantu Locs

After shampooing, conditioning, and slightly oiling your locs, make 1-2 inch sections of locs all over the head. Braid or twist each

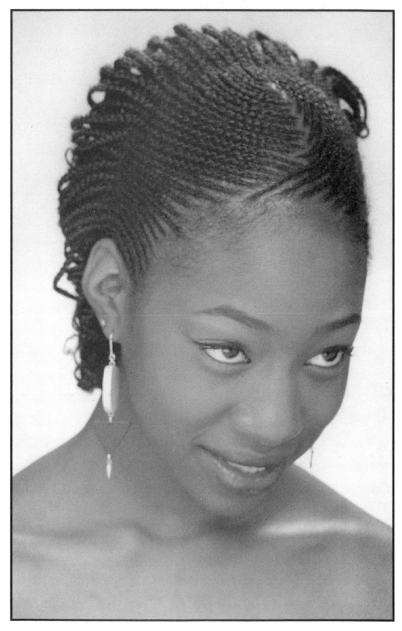

Ola's natural hair is cornrowed to the middle of her head. Individual braids adorn the base of the head.

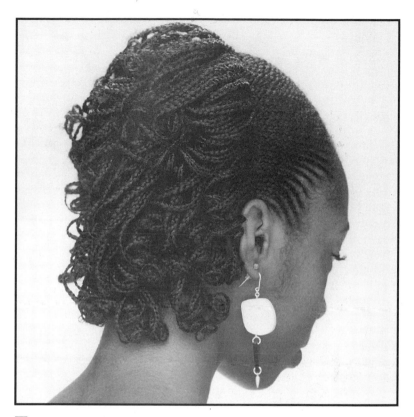

The ends of the cornrows were made into individual braids, then set on rollers to create gentle rolls or curls at the ends.

section together and then wrap them around to form a Bantu knot (see page 100). Let the hair dry 1-2 days and then take them out. According to the length of your hair you will be able to style them differently. For instance, a pony tail, Afrique roll (similar to a french roll), or because they're short, a texturized short loc look can be accomplished. Or, just let them hang and enjoy the feel of them.

Rod Set

This style works best with locs that are 10-12 inches long. After shampooing and conditioning the hair, apply a small amount of gel

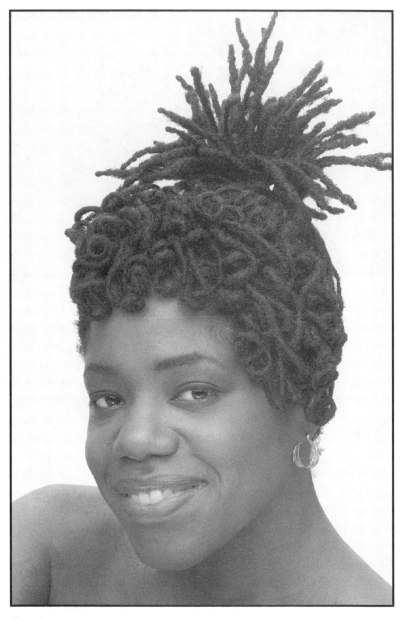

Lala's locs have been set on small rods to create tightly curled locs.

to one or two locs (depending on their thickness) and wrap them around a spiral rod. (These rods are available in professional beauty supply stores. Instruction for their usage is in the package.) Let the locs dry and remove the rods—you can let them hang or arrange them into something sophisticated or fun.

The thinner the diameter of the actual Loc, the more your styling options will increase. The thin Sister Locks boast of being able to achieve anything that relaxed hair can do, because they are so thin.

HAIR WRAPPING

Thread wrapping is a traditional art form that incorporates the use of thread to wrap braids or loose hair, to create hair sculptures. It is very popular on the west coast of Africa, in countries such as Nigeria and Senegal. African-American braiders have taken the process a few steps farther. They use synthetic hair (to make silky locs) and yarn (to make Genie Locs) instead of thread.

Genie Locs are created by braiding an extension fiber made of yarn into the natural hair, then wrapping the fiber around the braid to the desired length. This style can be worn for about three months. It is very durable, and can be washed and conditioned weekly. The process is the same for Silky Locs, as is their maintenance, but they last only two months. *Extreme caution must always be used when braiding and wrapping the hair.*

These are not styles for weak or damaged hair. Our hairlines tend to be weaker than any other part of the hair and scalp. This is the place where the first indication of real problems will surface. Sometimes the wrapping process can be painful. Take care. Although these styles are popular, your hair can easily become damaged if too much pressure is applied. Unfortunately, the only way you will be able to tell when you should not wrap your hair will be based on your experience. This technique is usually performed by

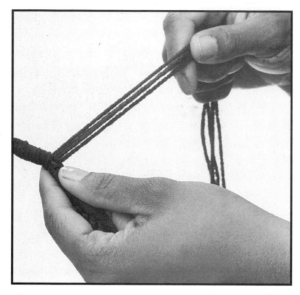

Acrylic yarn is wrapped around the braid. Start wrapping at the base of the scalp where the braid begins. (Synthetic hair can also be used to create Silky Locs.)

skilled professionals. Please do not attempt it if your hair is not healthy.

Start collecting your threads, needles, extension fibers, bobby pins and clips. Your vision has been expanded in the realm of adornment for natural hair. We have shared foundational techniques that with time and practice promise to reward you with creative expressions of your hair.

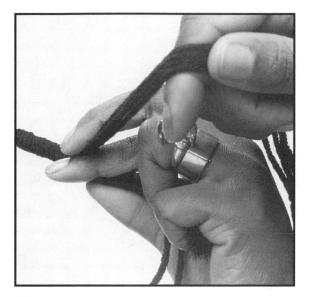

Continue wrapping the yarn down to the end of the braid.

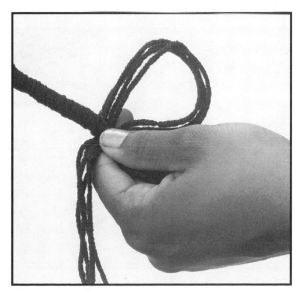

Fold the yarn, creating a loop.

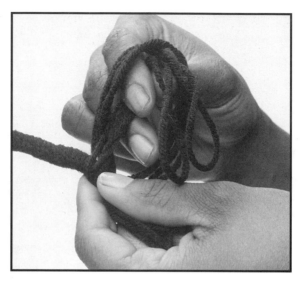

Take the hanging end of the yarn (end of the loop) and pull it back through the loop.

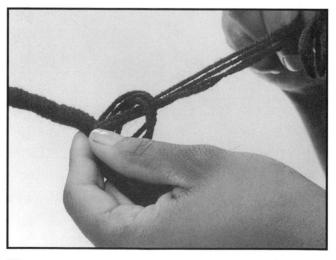

Pull the yarn through the loop and tighten. Tie a small knot on top of the slip knot and cut the yarn end.

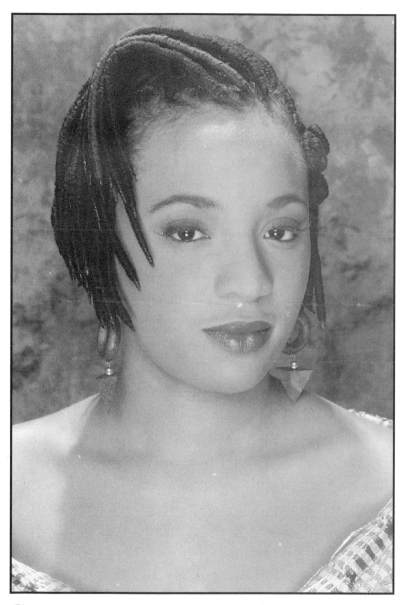

Genie Locs are the acrylic fiber version of silky locs. The yarn gives "locs" a sophisticated loc look. This style is durable and easy to maintain. With weekly shampooing and conditioning, it can last for three months. *(Stylists, Genique and Debra Hare-Bey)*

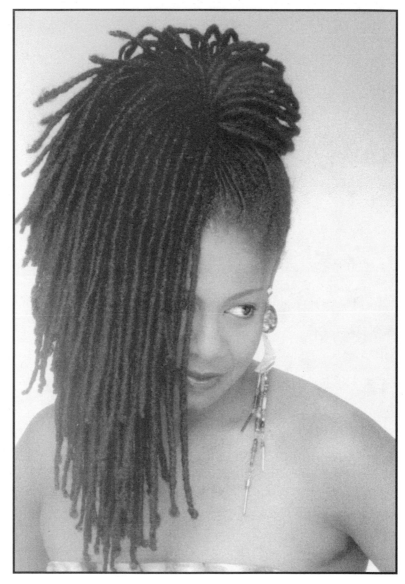

Phenomenal locs turn heads. Amma's locs always did and always will. *(Stylist, Tulani Kinard)*

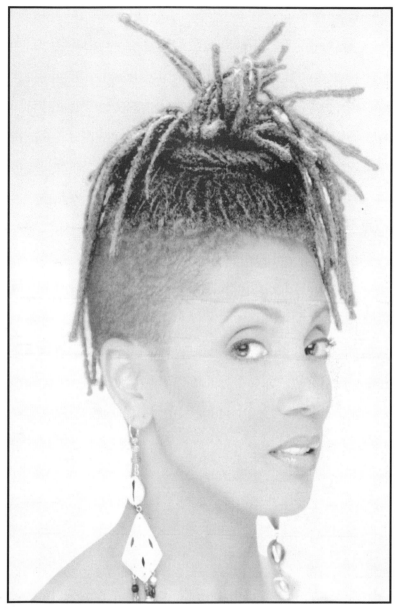

Karen's locs are fully matured. She wanted a different look without taking away all of her locs. Clear and committed to the natural aesthetic, she faded the sides and back of her hair. Her locs are styled to add height, and a sculptured beauty to her look. *(Stylist, Tulani Kinard)*

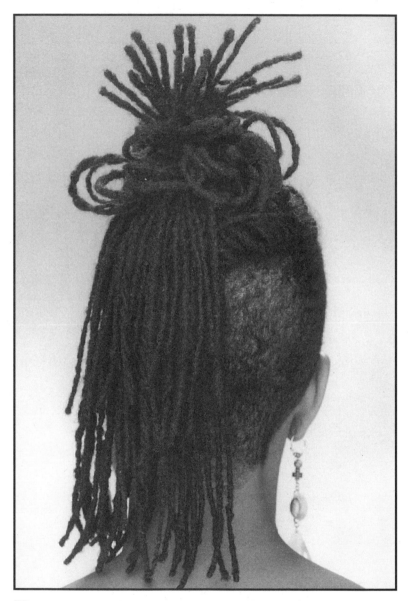

The back view of Karen's sculptured locs reveal a three-dimensional hair sculpture, the "Abebe (fan) Waterfall." This sculpture depicts the coolness of a breeze created by a fan, and the refreshment of the waterfall, both of which help to keep a "cool" head, enabling one to make good choices in life. *(Stylist, Tulani Kinard)*

I hope this chapter has whet your appetite, and made you want to discover and embrace the discipline of the art form. There are courses that are being offered all over the country. They are designed to support and train those who wish to expand their knowledge and skill level to a professional standard. Purchase a small, inexpensive camera and document your creations—you will grow from this.

The ancestral flow has just begun.

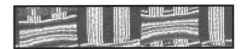

LITTLE BITS: CARING FOR
OUR CHILDREN'S HAIR

W

E ARE BLESSED to be in this era of growth and expansion of our consciousness about natural things. If you are reading this chapter with the intention of better caring for the young people in your life, it is with great joy that I share my experiences with you.

I remember being teased as a child by a couple of schoolmates whose hair was chemically straightened. They would sing, "It's going Afro! It's going Afro!" on days when the humidity caused by pressed hair to recoil into its natural state, while theirs stayed straight because their parents had used relaxers. My mother tried unsuccessfully to straighten my hair chemically. Fortunately, it was too soft to hold up to the abuse, and I wanted to wear my hair in an Afro anyway. Something had been awakened in my soul at a very impressionable age. In the late sixties, the Afro came in with the thunder of James Brown's "Say it loud, I'm Black and I'm proud." It was a time when young people could look around and see African-American women and men wearing their natural hair, and it felt wonderful. I wore my Afro proudly from middle school to adulthood. I was clear about my identity, and my hair was very important to me.

Children today are constantly evaluating and absorbing the images, lifestyles, and role models that their environment provides. They learn at an early age what they like to wear, and how they want their hair styled. So, the way we educate our children about their natural beauty from the very start of their lives is very important. Teaching them the significance and beauty of natural hair will lay a wonderful foundation for self-assured, strong, and culturally literate adults. Sure, it's easy to put a light perm in a child's hair. But now that you know what happens to their hair when you do, why put them through it? If convenience is your objective, it can be had—naturally.

If you decide to groom their hair you can plan on spending about twenty-five dollars per month on shampoo, conditioner, and moisturizing hair oils. The salon maintenance cost will vary depending on the maturity of the locs, and the age of the child. The salon grooming services should include a shampoo and deep conditioning treatment, moisturizing oil massage, and retwist. Baby locs (one week to six months) need to be groomed every three weeks. You could expect to pay anywhere from $35-$50 per session. When the locs mature the visits decrease to once a month, at a cost of $45-$65 per visit. The grooming price is largely based on the size of the child's head.

Most boys are making their first trip to the barber by age three, while by that age girls are getting acquainted with braids, barrettes, and bows. Times are changing.

We are starting to see more little boys wearing locs that have been cultivated from one and a half to two years old. I know there is a much more common occurrence of baby locs on little boys in urban areas than the suburbs or country provinces. But nevertheless, it's happening.

Cutting a girl's hair is not a commonplace thing. The general premise is to let it grow as long as it can for as long as it can. What is now inhibiting the healthy growth and development of their hair is the kiddy relaxers and the curly perms. The hair cutting that young girls are experiencing is largely based on cutting off the over-processed hair due to chemical damage.

INFANTS

An infant's hair is usually washed and groomed every time he or she is bathed. The soap used in the bath generally will also be used to shampoo the hair, unless there is some serious scalp problem and another solution is prescribed by the pediatrician. Cradle cap, for instance, is a common scalp condition that infants acquire. It is not contagious, and usually appears a week or two after birth. This condition appears because the sebaceous glands are overstimulated and become inflamed. This produces an unusual amount of sebum (oil) on the hair shaft. This oil settles on the skin, producing thick, scaly patches. Cradle cap is also common for adults, only it's called seborrhea and is often mistaken for dandruff. (Its similarities are the flaking scales that arise from an inflamed scalp.)

When treating your infant for this condition, *do not pick it, or try to rub the "cap" off* when shampooing the baby's hair. It will go away when the sebaceous glands and the skin's regeneration processes return to "normal." Some have to outgrow the condition, others have a brief bout and its like nothing ever happened. Shampoo the hair, massaging the scalp gently, then rinse. Towel-dry the baby's hair and scalp. Gently apply a little "Cradle Cap Ease" oil to the scalp area with your fingertips, but avoid touching the fontanelle (the soft spot at the top of the skull). Please observe your baby's reaction to this mixture. If it is adverse, stop using it. Even though this is 100 percent natural, "different strokes for different folks" still applies. Use the oil mixture daily for three weeks until the cradle cap goes away. If it has not gone away, discontinue use and have a doctor examine your child.

CRADLE CAP EASE OIL

1 drop eucalyptus oil*
½ drop chamomile oil
3 tablespoons sweet almond oil

Mix oils. (Essential oils must be mixed in a base vegetable oil when they are to be applied directly to the skin.) Funnel the mixture into a small brown bottle, close tightly, and store in a cool, dark location.

THE RIGHT SHAMPOO FOR YOUR CHILD

Any shampoo that is pH-balanced and moisturizing, even if it's for dry and damaged hair, is generally a good choice. These shampoos are designed to replenish the moisture in the hair shaft. Up to the age of three to four years old, baby shampoo should still be effective, unless you are applying heavy pomades, greases, and oils to the child's head as part of their grooming regimen. If this is the case, then there's no need for you to dilute the shampoo. With the dust and debris from the air and all that the grease and oil would attract, the cleansing power of the shampoo would be needed. Instead of shampooing their hair two to three times as you would an adult, do it one time full-strength, or dilute the shampoo with water at a fifty-fifty ratio and shampoo the hair twice. Follow this mode of thinking until the age of six years old. Then start decreasing the dilution ratio from fifty–fifty to 75 percent shampoo to 25 percent water.

A good conditioner should be used after each shampoo. As a rule, choose a conditioner based upon the texture and thickness (or thinness) of the child's hair. Decrease the amount suggested for an

---

* You should be able to find any of these ingredients at a well-stocked, neighborhood health-food store that carries essential oils.

adult by half. Careful observation of the texture, luster, and body of the hair will guide you to just the right amount needed to use (keep in mind a drop the size of a quarter or if need be a dime is quite often more than enough).

Most conditioners will say for fine hair, for dry hair, for normal hair—observe the condition of their hair and choose accordingly.

A weekly regimen of washing and conditioning your child's hair, along with a diet that is packed with green, leafy vegetables and fiber, is the best way to cultivate a healthy head of hair for your little one. This regimen is good for both boys and girls. If the boys have closely cropped haircuts, after shampooing the hair, follow up by applying a light oil (see page 89), brushing, and/or combing the hair.

FOR GIRLS, NO-TRAUMA DRAMA: THE COMB-OUT

After shampooing and conditioning, separate the hair into small sections according to the thickness and length of your daughter's hair—deal with what feels comfortable for you to manage. Take a small section of the hair, holding it firmly at the scalp; using a wide-toothed comb, gently comb through the ends of the hair. Gradually work your way down, combing upward and out, until you reach the scalp. You should be able to pull the comb through the section gently without popping the hair shaft out of the scalp.

Separate the finished section into two halves and twist them together. Then go on to the next section. After combing through each section, take a blow dryer and set the controls to the lowest setting. Comb through each section with the blow dryer the same way you combed through the hair with the wide-toothed comb. Upon completion, the hair is ready to be styled. A light moisturizing oil may be applied to the scalp and hair at this point. If you are preparing the child's hair to be braided by a natural-hair-care specialist, ask if they want any oils applied to the hair prior to the appointment.

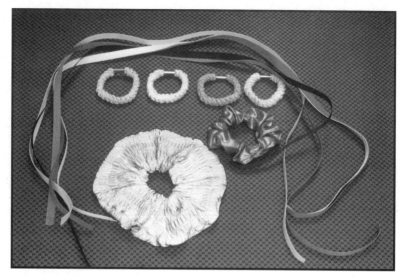

Various adornments which can be used to tie back your braids.

When styling, do not use rubber bands or other types of adornments (clips, combs, barrettes, bubbles) that would pull the hair together too tightly.

Choose hairstyles that don't require tight braiding. Too much tension on the scalp will cause pain, sores, and in severe cases, hair loss. Single plaits and twists are very nice styles for toddlers. Ribbons are better to use than rubber bands to hold the hair in place. At the end of the first week, the hair should be shampooed and conditioned. A light moisturizing hair oil should be applied daily or as often as needed, depending on the natural hair type. When braids are removed, the hair should be shampooed, conditioned, dried, combed, and brushed again, in preparation for the next style. The only reason a child's hair should not be combed and brushed on a "regular" basis is because they have locs, braids, or other temporary styles.

As the hair grows in length and thickness, a variation of natural and extension styles will aid growth and development of the hair by providing different types of stimulation to the scalp. As long as your child's natural hair is at least three inches long, cornrows, individual braids, and twisted styles can be attained. The regular braiding of a child's hair will not allow her to acquire a sensitive scalp, generally due to lack of combing and brushing. Between the ages of four and ten, their hair should be braided regularly—every two to three weeks. At the time that the braid style moves to a three-week span, synthetic extensions can be introduced to hold the hairstyle in place, protecting it from fraying and coming out of the braids. Braid one small braid of the extension into her hair; this will be an overnight test strand to determine if the skin shows an allergic reaction to the synthetic fiber.

These natural styles can last a week or longer, depending on the skill level of the stylist—you!

Natural, individual braids and twists are two lovely looks that hold up through shampooing. Older children can have their hair set on curling rods (air-drying is best), or Bantu knots, to achieve a

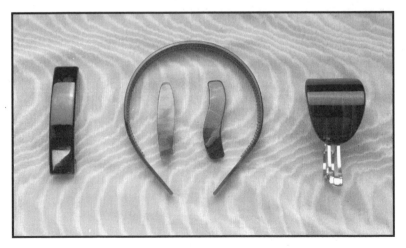

These hair ornaments are safe to use on your child's hair. They will not put any damaging tension on the hair or scalp. They may be used on natural hair, braids, locs, and even chemically straightened hair.

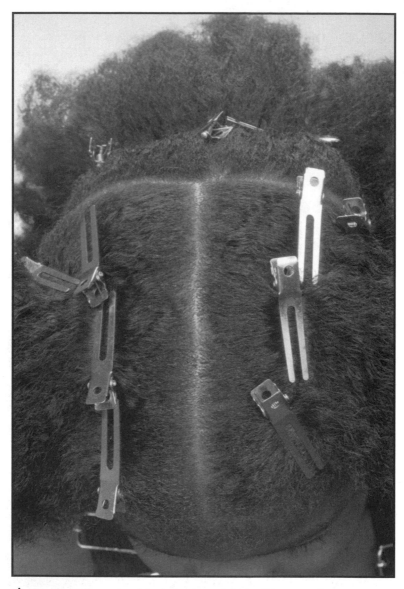

Avion is creating a simple style for Sinead that will last a week. Part the hair, then clip the hair not being worked on with a large duck clip.

very curly style for variation during the two-week span of time the braids last. During the two weeks the hair should only be washed and conditioned at the end of the first week. This would be the best time to Bantu-knot, or to set the style on small rods.

Cornrows, braided with the correct tension on the scalp, have served for centuries as a classic style to aid in scalp stimulation and hair growth.

After the third or fourth stitch has been established, have the child place his or her finger at the base of the cornrow and pull the base forward. What will happen is while the cornrow is being braided, the pull forward is creating an opposing tension so when the cornrow is completed and the finger removed, a balanced tension in the braid will exist that will be comfortable yet secure.

The younger the child (three to four years old), the larger the braids should be. The older the child (five to nine years old), the smaller the braids. In both cases there is an exception—taking into

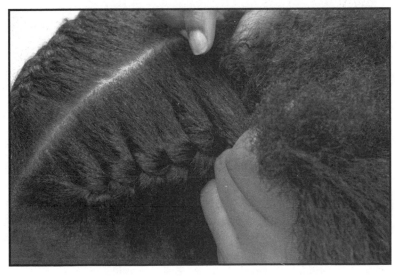

Be careful not to apply too much pressure or tension on the hairline as you are braiding your child's hair. As a rule of thumb, if your child is in discomfort while having their hair braided, and after the style is completed they are still experiencing the discomfort, then take it out.

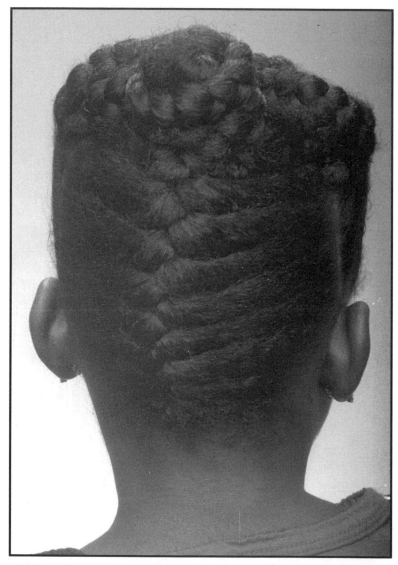

This is a simple but elegant style that if covered with a cotton scarf at night, will look beautiful throughout the week. *(Stylist, Avion Julien)*

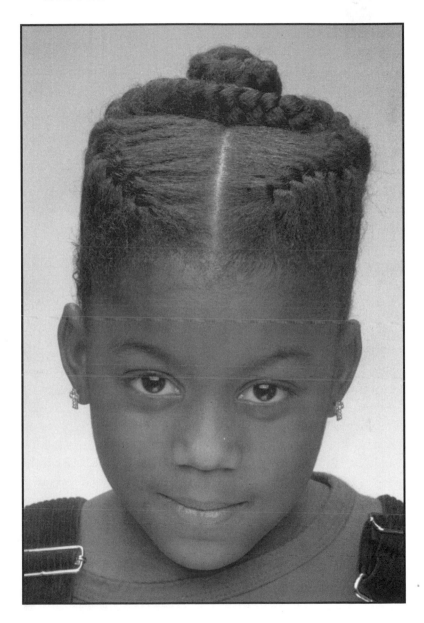

account the temperament of your child. If you have a child who is very active, speed and proficiency in styling are of the utmost importance. Having someone read a story, or showing a good children's video, while you're styling the child's hair will make the process a lot easier.

Depending on the size of the cornrows, they may be kept in for one day, or up to a week. These braids rest on the scalp and are easy to redo fairly quickly—particularly important if you have a toddler who has "discovered" his or her legs.

As the child gets older (seven to ten years old), styles may be kept in a little longer—three to four weeks at a time. Preteens to teenagers can begin to look forward to more elaborate styles, which can stay in up to four to six weeks at a time.

I cannot stress enough the importance of a weekly, or at minimum biweekly, shampooing and conditioning regimen, with the use of a light moisturizing hair oil to aid in the rejuvenation and growth process. By the time a child reaches four years of age, her scalp should have sufficiently developed to support the additional weight of extension hair. I recommend that any extension styling be done by a licensed natural-hair-care specialist if possible. I cannot begin to count the time I have witnessed little girls living out their parents' "mo' hair" syndrome, walking around with extension braids all the way down their backs. This styling is very detrimental to the healthy growth and development of the child's hair. Children between the ages of five and nine should not have extensions that go below the nape of the neck, or at best their outer shoulders. That is more than enough length to create different styles. I absolutely do not recommend large Casamas braids for them. The amount of extension hair required to create these styles is too heavy for hanging or cornrow braids. As a rule, extensions should be used to hold/support their natural hair in a cornrow. For single braids, the extension hair used should not exceed the amount of natural hair. A fifty-fifty ratio is not always possible, due to breakage, thinness, and chemical damage. These are the exception to the rule.

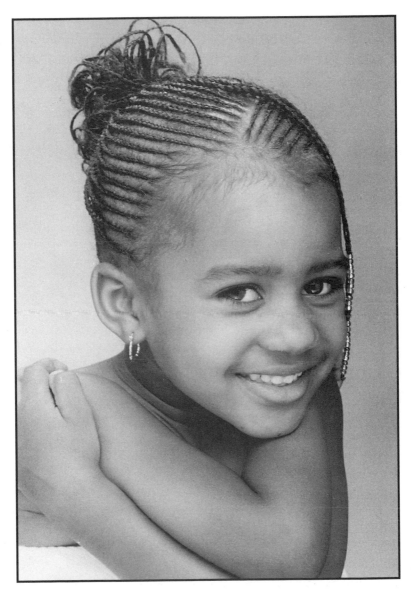

Osaremi has had her natural hair cornrowed into a style that will last two to three weeks (at the discretion of her mom). The cornrows were braided away from her face. Her hairline was not disturbed: she still has lanugo hair around her face. It is important not to try to pull the soft, fine hair up into the corn-row when braiding. This will cause damage to the hairline.

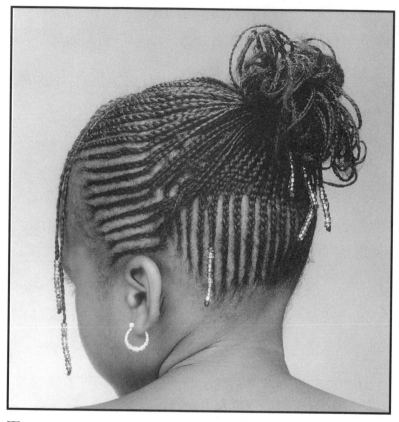

The same care must be observed when braiding the back of the hair. Os-aremi's cornrows have been braided up and away from the nape of her neck with single braids in the middle of her head to add depth and thickness to the "ponytail." A few glass beads provide slight ornamentation that will not clash with any bows or ribbons that might be added at another time. *(Stylist, Avion Julien)*

NO PAIN . . . NO PAIN

Any level of pain is your signal to stop the braiding process. If the pain is not present during, but appears soon after the style is completed, take the braids out immediately. It's not natural for this to occur. Little red pustule bumps, migraine-type headaches, the

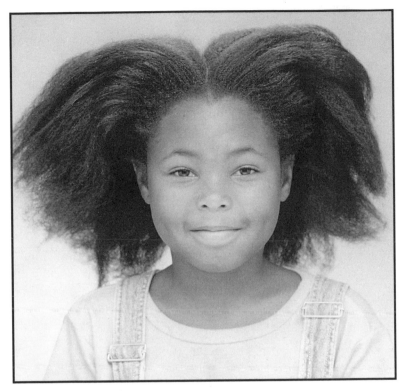

Alexzandria's natural hair is about eight to ten inches long in various places all over her head. Her hair has been groomed exclusively with Nu Ade moisturizing hair lotion for the past three years.

loss of hair follicles, even permanent hair loss in the area, can all result from the experience. Not to mention the pain, which may create a phobia in your child about having her hair braided. The braid styles created for this age should not take any longer than one or two hours to complete, and should not be left in any longer than two weeks at a time.

Both time and money are invested, but the equity is a beautiful, healthy head of hair, along with a strong cultural aesthetic that will support your children to and throughout adulthood.

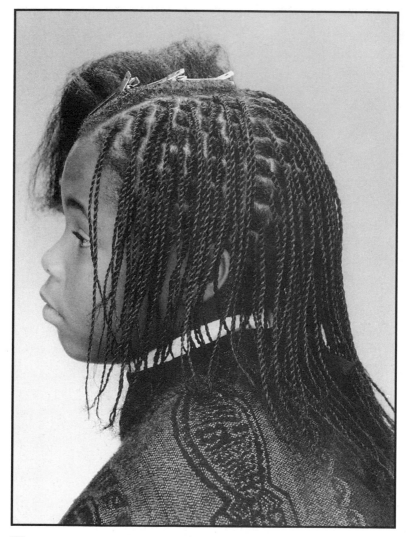

The hair is parted in equal sections all over her head and a two-stranded twist is done in each sectioned part.

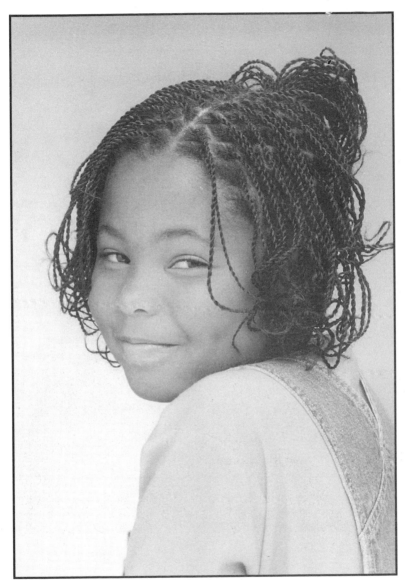

The natural twists are curled up on the ends and styled in one of the many styles that Alexzandria likes to wear. This style takes two hours to complete and lasts up to two months. *(Stylist, Avion Julien)*

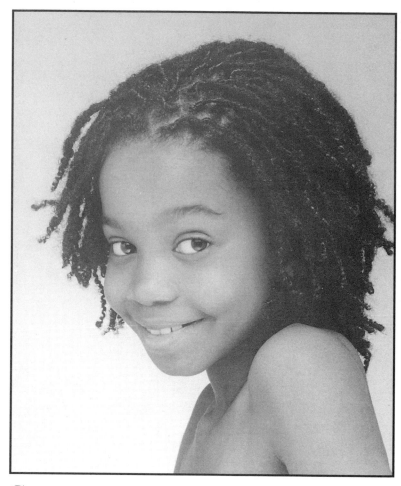

Gabriell's locs were started as two-stranded twists (like Alexzandria's hair). The twists were never taken out. After weekly grooming sessions her hair began to loc after three months. The locs are seven months old.

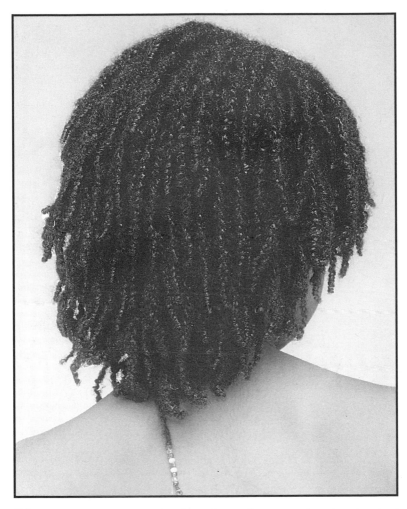

Gabriell's hair is shampooed and conditioned every week and moisturized with Nu Crown moisturizing hair oil. Her locs are retwisted once a month.

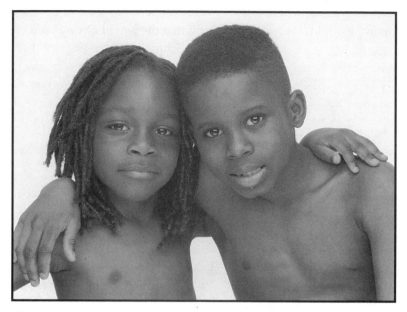

Alade with a closely cropped haircut and Olatunde with groomed, mature locs exemplify the spectrum of styles young boys are wearing.

IT'S A LOC!

Locs are a natural way to cultivate a healthy head of hair. They may be started at any age. As soon as the baby's hair is able to stay entwined, you may begin. I recommend waiting until the lanugo hair disappears before beginning locs. By the age of five, the texture of the hair will have changed, and will be closer to the child's mature hair texture. Once the locking process has begun, whoever is going to be responsible for the grooming (parent or "loctician") must pay particular attention to keeping the shaft of the locs clean after they are formed. Dust and debris cling to the hair, and you know children are really active—rolling on the floor, playing outside, etc. So little cotton or silk hats that are able to cover the entire head can help to keep dust out while letting the hair "breathe."

Keeping the little one's head groomed is another level of commitment. I would strongly recommend that the parent or care provider become proficient in grooming techniques (see page 131 on proper grooming techniques) for those times when you cannot keep a loctician appointment. Adults can slide. Children, because of their active lifestyles, really shouldn't.

HELPING OUR SONS SHINE

For the first time in almost a generation, our men are wearing long, styled, natural hair. Isn't it wonderful? Although this is basically a guide for black women, I feel confident in saying we are the caretakers of most of those beautiful male heads. My particular concern is to address our young men and boys, who are wearing these styles without direction. Most of them don't have a clue as to how to groom their hair. Please share the information in this book with your young men. If you are the one responsible for any of those heads, make sure you give their hair the same amount of attention that you would give your own. Train them well. I also encourage you to share this book with the men you know who are taking care of their own natural hair, as well as their children's. I really want to see young men with beautifully groomed, natural hair. It is a powerful statement of cultural consciousness, and manhood.

In 1990, I did several lectures with Leasa Farrar-Fortune, who is an educational specialist at the National Museum of African Art. She showed slides of young, South African men in the 1700s. Their haircuts incorporated tribal symbols that spoke to their stature in the community and things that were important to them. They were very much like the designer cuts we see today on the heads of our young men.

Take time to sow positive, spiritual, cultural, historical, family-oriented, community-concerned seeds into their crowns. While you are locking their hair you are also opening their minds—that's your "charge to keep."

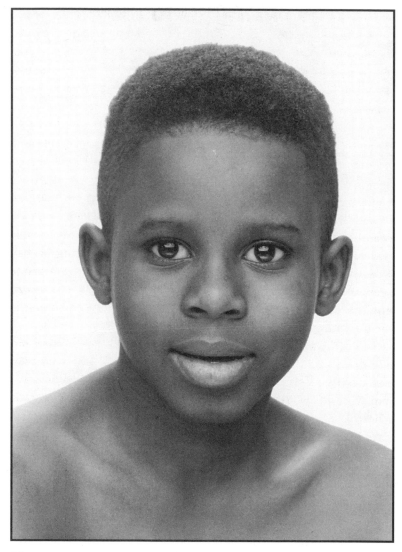

Closely cropped haircuts for little boys are very easy to maintain. Alade cares for his hair by oiling his scalp as needed and brushing his hair every day.

FROM ONE MOTHER TO ANOTHER

If locking your child's hair is not a cultural way of life for you, then careful consideration should be given to the time commitment you will have to make if you choose this path. My son, Alade, came to me when he was six years old, begging me to start locking his hair. All of my immediate family members have locs. I comb-twisted his hair, and he went about his business living the life of a six-year-old boy. Well, three days later, half of the twists were gone, and the other half looked terrible. With my schedule, I was doing well if he made it to the barber every three weeks. Needless to say, we really could not have our son walking around with his head like that, and I was not willing to comb-twist his hair every two days. I knew he would not be able to handle having his hair retwisted so much, and I was not going to contract our loctitian to keep up with his grooming needs. We made an agreement to wait until he was eleven years old, so he would be able to take part in the grooming of his locs.

My daughter, Sakeenah, has worn natural hairstyles all her life, and at the age of ten we started her locs. They began as two-stranded twists with tiny glass beads on the ends. She had no problem with her peers at school, until her hair really started to lock. The more her hair locked, the more static she received. She endured cultural racism, which at first was very hard for her to understand. What do I mean by cultural racism? It is when members of your own race discriminate against you and harass you because of a cultural belief that is not their own. Her peers did not understand why she would want to wear locs instead of a perm. At eleven, twelve, and thirteen years of age, almost all of her school peers had chemical relaxers in their hair. She put up with the kind of abuse that one would expect from someone totally ignorant of our culture and full of hate for our people. However, self-hatred tends to run deep in our community, and children are often the conveyors of just how far we have really come. She endured these insults in silence for a long time, wondering how her peers could say the things they were saying. Many of the derogatory things

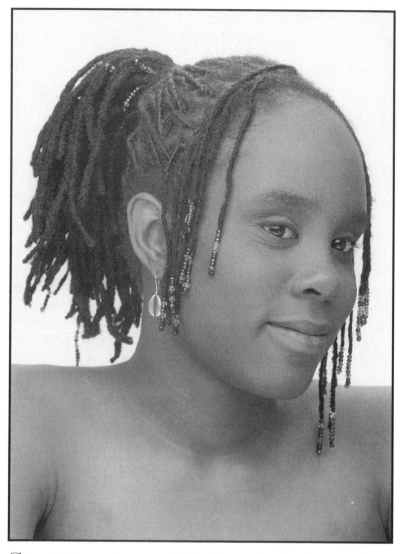

Sakeenah's locs are three years old. She likes wearing them in a ponytail with bangs hanging in the front.

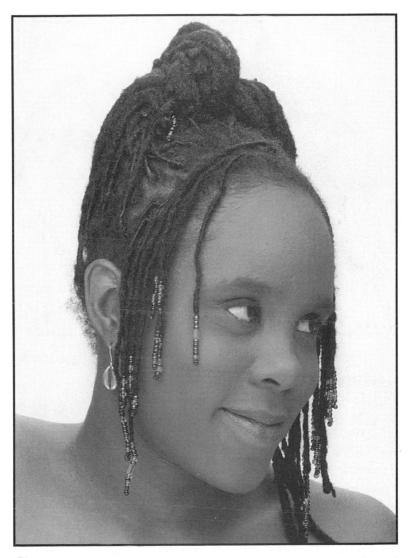

Sakeenah's locs have been gathered together and styled to create a sculptured crown, with beaded locs cascading on either side of her face.

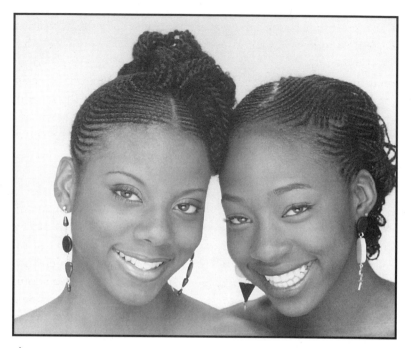

Arlene and Ola love wearing their hair in natural cornrows. These styles last two months with weekly shampooing and conditioning. Their braided ends were curled to add just the right finishing touch. *(Stylist, Nicole James)*

they said were based upon them thinking she was a Rastafarian because her hair was locked. Years of negative media images of Rastafarians color our imaginations. They've been portrayed as scruffy, marijuana-smoking anarchists who seek to undermine all of what society holds dear. Every day we affirmed her beauty, and discussed the truth about natural hair.

I had to educate her about chemical straighteners, and the reasons why people choose to apply these products to their hair. She began to notice her classmates' hair thinning. She concluded that the damage she witnessed was caused by chemical straighteners. Somebody once said that knowledge is power. Sakeenah's knowledge about natural hair care enabled her to take a nonconfrontational posture that stood the test of time. Eventually the harassment ceased. Soon her classmates were commenting on how much they liked her beads. They asked how long it would take them to get their hair done like hers. Sakeenah has never had the experience of having her hair burned with a straightening comb, nor the burning scalp sensation from a chemical straightener. She has known the beauty of her natural hair from birth. Children must see themselves, and be exposed to those who reflect a standard of beauty that embraces who they are.

We now have a great opportunity to educate our young people. There are magazines that are committed to promoting a natural Afrocentric style of wearing our hair, including *Braids and Beauty, Sophisticate's Black Hair,* and *Essence,* just to name a few. Most of the styles are for adults, but buy them for your home to help encourage a natural Afrocentric aesthetic in your child's life. You should take your children and young people to museums that exhibit African art. Discover the beauty and power that exists in the sculptures, textiles, and jewelry. The artistic expression of African sculptors demonstrates the spiritual and ancestral omnipresence of God throughout African culture. Every home should have books like *Africa Adorned* by Angela Fisher. It is a wonderful photojournalistic tour of many different countries and cultures in Africa.

Children and teenagers must know that their heads are a sacred place. They should be filled not only with knowledge and love of self, but also with our history as a people, respect for our ancestors, respect for living elders, each other, nature, and our community. If a natural head of hair is cultivated and adorned to reflect our historical lineage, many of the problems we face in raising our children, in a society filled with violence and negative influences, will be solved.

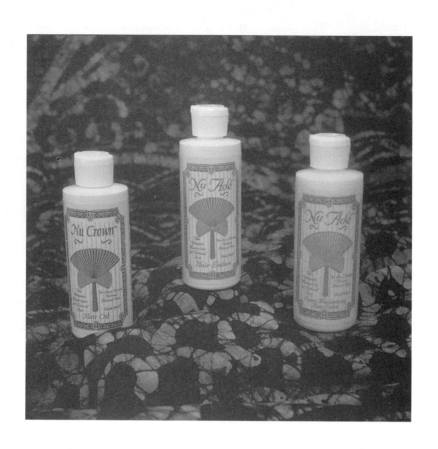

TULANI PROUDLY PRESENTS:

ORDER FORM INFORMATION

Name

Address

City

State

Zip

Phone

Nu Crown Hair Oil stimulates the follicles and leaves a sheen on the hair that reflects health and beauty. The oil is light, deep penetrating, and absorbs quickly into the scalp and skin.

2 oz. $4.00 / 4 oz. $8.50 / 8 oz. $17.00

Nu Ade Moisturizing Hair Lotion has a special moisturizing formula which helps to lock in moisture and strengthen the hair. It also provides a soothing coolness for the irritated scalp.

2 oz. $6.00 / 4 oz. $13.00 / 8 oz. $25.00

Nu Ade Super Moist Hair Lotion is the ultimate moisturizer for dry, damaged, lifeless hair. This product penetrates the scalp and hair shaft, leaving the hair soft, supple, and well conditioned.

2 oz. $7.00 / 4 oz. $16.75 / 8 oz. $27.00

All orders are payable by money order, certified check, American Express, Visa, or Mastercard. These products are aromatherapeutic; they are also available without scents.

Please send all orders to:

Nu Ade Enterprises

591 Vanderbilt Avenue

Suite 208

Brooklyn, NY 11238

(718) 604-3001